Treatment planning in primary dental care

Oxford University Press makes no representation, express or implied, that the drug dosages in this book are correct. Readers must therefore always check the product information and clinical procedures with the most up to date published product information and data sheets provided by the manufacturers and the most recent codes of conduct and safety regulations. The authors and the publishers do not accept responsibility or legal liability for any errors in the text or for the misuse or misapplication of material in this work.

Treatment planning in primary dental care

Ann C. Shearer

Consultant in Restorative Dentistry, Dundee Dental Hospital, Dundee, UK

Anthony C. Mellor

Senior Lecturer in Primary Dental Care, University Dental Hospital of Manchester, UK

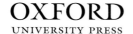

OXFORD

UNIVERSITY PRESS

OXFORD
UNIVERSITY PRESS

Great Clarendon Street, Oxford OX2 6DP

Oxford University Press is a department of the University of Oxford.
It furthers the University's objective of excellence in research, scholarship,
and education by publishing worldwide in

Oxford New York
Auckland Bangkok Buenos Aires Cape Town Chennai
Dar es Salaam Delhi Hong Kong Istanbul Karachi Kolkata
Kuala Lumpur Madrid Melbourne Mexico City Mumbai Nairobi
São Paulo Shanghai Taipei Tokyo Toronto

Oxford is a registered trade mark of Oxford University Press
in the UK and in certain other countries

Published in the United States
by Oxford University Press Inc., New York

A catalogue record for this title is available from the British Library

ISBN 0 19 850895 6

10 9 8 7 6 5 4 3 2 1

Typeset by Newgen Imaging Systems (P) Ltd., Chennai, India
Printed in Italy on acid-free paper by Legoprint

Contents

1 Principles of planning care

INTRODUCTION

The principles of planning dental care would appear to be very simple. Information is gathered from the patient, the patient is examined, the dentist considers the possible treatment options, and then the patient and the dentist decide together on the most suitable way forward.

However, as with most facets of life, it is not quite that simple. There are many aspects that need to be considered in each case and the aim of this book is to lay down a blueprint that students and practitioners can follow.

We are not aiming to be prescriptive, as we realise that each case is different. What we will do is to provide a framework on which any case can be built. In this book we will presume that all the patients will be new patients to the student or practitioner and therefore no information will be assumed.

IS ANY CASE SIMPLE?

It may be that some cases will not need the range of planning that others will. However, we hope to help you recognise which cases are simple and which are more complex. For example, a patient presenting for the replacement of an anterior crown may seem a simple case, but there are factors such as the occlusal relationship or the presence of parafunctional habits which may make the treatment planning stage more lengthy.

INTEGRATING CARE IN RESTORATIVE DENTISTRY

Undergraduate dental students are taught the various aspects of restorative dentistry by teachers with expertise in operative dentistry, endodontics, periodontics, prosthodontics and biomaterial science. These subjects are usually taught by individual units or departments with varying levels of integration. However, in the latter part of the course, students may practise integrated or comprehensive restorative care for their patients, bringing together the knowledge they have gained in the various restorative disciplines. This approach more accurately simulates the care provided in general dental practice and is therefore essential preparation for the practitioner.

HOW TO PLAN DENTAL CARE

The process of planning care begins with collecting information which will lead to a diagnosis. This is fundamental to the success of the process. If the correct diagnosis is not reached, then the appropriate treatment will not necessarily be prescribed. Some students and practitioners are so keen to get on with the treatment that they forget about the diagnosis. Listing the diagnoses e.g. caries, chronic periodontitis, will provide the basis of the treatment plan and also the treatment priorities.

LISTENING SKILLS

The importance of listening skills to a dentist cannot be overestimated. The patient is the consumer of your dental skills and has a right to expect that their views will be heard and properly considered. Listening skills are complemented by questioning skills and by giving the patient time to think and answer. Where there is a lot of information to consider, this process may take a number of visits. Written as well as verbal information will need to be given to the patient to allow them to decide what treatment they will accept.

In the next chapter, the information you need to collect for successful treatment planning will be considered.

2 Gathering information

INTRODUCTION

First impressions are vital in any professional situation. If you can make a good impression at the first visit then this will start to build the trust that is essential in a successful dentist–patient relationship. In a practice situation, the receptionist and dental nurse also play an important role in presenting the image of an efficient, caring practice.

A few basic points should be borne in mind:
- Try to ensure that you see the patient on time.
- Greet the patient when they enter and introduce yourself.
- Smile and try to make the patient feel at ease.
- Invite the patient to sit in the dental chair and make sure that they are comfortable.

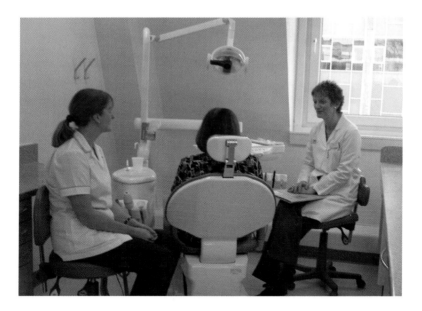

Figure 2.1 Taking a history.

- Seat yourself facing the patient, preferably at the same level.
- Make eye contact with the patient during your conversation.

You will need to make notes, but do not write while the patient is talking as this gives the impression you are not paying attention (fig. 2.1).

You are then ready to start taking the patient history. This is divided into four sections:

- History of the presenting complaint (if any)
- Medical history
- Dental history
- Social history.

HISTORY OF THE PRESENTING COMPLAINT

We have assumed that the patient is a new patient to you. It is wise to start with a general question such as 'What can we do for you today?'. An open question like this gives the patient the opportunity to set the agenda for the visit and imparts a certain amount of control.

The patient may not be having any problems and simply request a routine examination. However, if there is a problem then this needs to be explored by more probing questions. We must ask the patient:

- To describe the problem in their own words. If they have pain, then what type of pain is it? Is it a shooting pain, a throbbing pain, or just a dull ache? Does it radiate to other areas? Has this problem occurred previously?

- The duration of the problem. How long has the problem been there? Is it constant or intermittent in nature and is it stable or worsening?
- The severity of the problem. Is the patient able to function normally? Can they eat or brush their teeth? Does the pain disturb sleep?
- About any exacerbating or relieving factors. Is it worse with any stimuli such as heat or pressure? If analgesics have been taken, were they totally or partially effective?
- About any previous treatment. Has the patient attended another dentist or their general medical practitioner? Has any treatment been carried out or any drugs prescribed?

These initial questions will usually give you an idea of the probable nature of the problem. The next phase is to elucidate the patient's medical history.

THE MEDICAL HISTORY

Structured questions will lead to a clear idea of the patient's medical status. Some practices ask the patient to complete a written medical history questionnaire in the waiting area prior to being seen. This can then be read by the dentist and any points clarified.

If you are taking a verbal medical history, it is wise to preface any questions with a simple explanatory introduction such as 'I now need to go over your medical history for our records'. This can be followed by a general question such as 'Are you generally fit and well?'. This allows the patient to lead the process and describe in their terms any medical problems they have.

For the purposes of dental treatment we then need to ask specifically about any history of:

- Heart disease or circulatory problems e.g. coronary artery disease, hypertension or stroke.
- Chest or lung disease e.g. bronchitis, asthma, emphysema.
- Liver diseases e.g. jaundice, hepatitis.
- Rheumatic fever.
- Diabetes – insulin-controlled, drug-controlled or diet-controlled.
- Epilepsy.
- Allergic reactions to any drugs. We are especially interested in any reactions to antibiotics, as these are the most common drugs that we are likely to prescribe to a patient. Patients who say that they are allergic to a drug should be questioned further to establish the nature of the allergy. Those who have had a rash following the administration of a drug are likely to have a true allergy. Other patients who say they are allergic have often had symptoms of nausea or other gastrointestinal upset. This is unlikely to be a true allergy but it does indicate intolerance and the drug in question should be avoided if possible.

- Current drugs (tablets or medication) prescribed by their doctor. The names and daily dosage of all drugs should be noted, consulting the *Dental Practitioner's Formulary* (DPF) or the *Monthly Index of Medical Specialties* (MIMS) for clarification if necessary. This should include creams and inhalers which some patients do not consider to be drugs. If you just ask about tablets, you may miss something significant. For example, patients who have used a steroid cream regularly for a skin condition may have adrenal suppression.
- Bleeding disorders. This question should be phrased in a general way – 'Do you have any history of excessive bleeding when you cut yourself or anything like that?'. If a patient reports excessive bleeding after dental extractions, this should be explored. Did it just happen on one occasion or is this a regular occurrence? If it is the latter, this requires a preoperative blood test if extractions are planned. Asking about any other operations that the patient has undergone may be of use. If a patient has had a tonsillectomy without consequence then it is unlikely they have a bleeding diathesis.
- Any medical treatment in the past three months. This is a back-up question to draw out any other medical conditions that may be of significance.

Some medical history questionnaires ask specifically about HIV or AIDS status. This is not necessary as all patients should be treated as potentially infectious and appropriate cross-infection procedures should be in place. Many HIV/AIDS patients will volunteer the information about their infection but some may not, often as a result of being refused treatment previously.

THE DENTAL HISTORY

You want to assess the patient's attitude to dentistry as well as their past dental experiences, as this may influence the way care is provided and what treatment options are possible.

Patient attitudes to dentistry

Is the patient a regular dental attender? When was the last dental attendance? What treatment was carried out then? How do they feel about coming to the dentist? Have they had any problems with dental treatment in the past? These simple questions will allow the patient to express their opinions as well as any concerns or fears that they have about dentistry.

You can evaluate a patient's level of anxiety using both *qualitative* and *quantitative* measures. The qualitative measures are from observation and from the history. Does the patient appear nervous; are there signs of shaking, sweating or even crying? Patients who are nervous often talk incessantly while others avoid eye contact. Increased dental anxiety is associated with irregular dental attendance. Your receptionist or dental nurse can often warn you of patients with extreme anxiety, either from when they arrange an appointment or from their appearance on presentation.

Quantitative measures can be used to objectively measure dental anxiety. The most well known scale is the Corah Dental Anxiety Scale which has been modified recently to include a question on attitudes to local anaesthesia (fig. 2.2). Other established scales are the Structured Interview for Assessing Dental Fear (SIADF), the State–Trait Anxiety Inventory (STAI) and the Dental Fear Survey.

1. If you went to your dentist for TREATMENT TOMORROW, how would you feel?

☐	☐	☐	☐	☐
Not Anxious	Slightly Anxious	Fairly Anxious	Very Anxious	Extremely Anxious

2. If you were sitting in the WAITING ROOM (waiting for treatment), how would you feel?

☐	☐	☐	☐	☐
Not Anxious	Slightly Anxious	Fairly Anxious	Very Anxious	Extremely Anxious

3. If you were about to have a TOOTH DRILLED, how would you feel?

☐	☐	☐	☐	☐
Not Anxious	Slightly Anxious	Fairly Anxious	Very Anxious	Extremely Anxious

4. If you were about to have your teeth SCALED AND POLISHED, how would you feel?

☐	☐	☐	☐	☐
Not Anxious	Slightly Anxious	Fairly Anxious	Very Anxious	Extremely Anxious

5. If you were about to have a LOCAL ANAESTHETIC INJECTION in your gum above an upper back tooth, how would you feel?

☐	☐	☐	☐	☐
Not Anxious	Slightly Anxious	Fairly Anxious	Very Anxious	Extremely Anxious

Each item is scored as follows: *Not anxious* = 1
Slightly anxious = 2
Fairly anxious = 3
Very anxious = 4
Extremely anxious = 5

Total score is a sum of all five items, range 5–25

Figure 2.2 The Modified Dental Anxiety Scale (Humphris *et al.* 1995).

Past dental experiences

Before examining the patient's mouth, it is useful to establish what sort of treatment they have had previously and under what conditions. What types of treatment has the patient undergone e.g. fillings, extractions, etc.? Has the patient had treatment under local anaesthesia, under local anaesthesia with sedation or under general anaesthesia? Has the patient any preferences in terms of treatment? An increasing number of patients are concerned about the possible toxic effects of mercury in amalgam and are requesting alternative materials.

THE SOCIAL HISTORY

The social conditions under which a patient lives may have a bearing on their general or dental health. Caring for a sick partner or being under pressure at work are both situations that can be stressful. The link between stress and disease is well known and has been described as the stress–disease model (fig. 2.3).

Understanding your patient's social conditions will help you to plan treatment in a way that will fit in with the rest of their life. For example, their availability for treatment may be limited by work or home commitments or by travel difficulties. Therefore, you might try to complete treatment in a small number of long treatment sessions rather than a larger number of shorter treatment sessions.

Tobacco and alcohol consumption

The relationship between smoking and periodontal disease is well established and recently a link between periodontal disease and cardiovascular disease has been described. In addition, smoking has been described as a major factor in the prevalence of dry socket following extractions and is a contraindicator for the provision of endosseous implants. It is therefore highly relevant to know if the patient smokes and to what extent.

Excessive alcohol consumption can be associated with liver damage. This may lead to increased bleeding tendencies after extractions or intolerance to

---

Stress-disease model

Social environment/social circumstances → psychological/emotional states → physiological processes → disease/susceptibility to disease

(Locker 1989)

Figure 2.3 Stress-disease model.

certain drugs. A gentle enquiry into whether a patient drinks alcohol, and if so to what extent, is therefore a vital part of the social history.

THE EXAMINATION

Having completed the history, explain to the patient that an examination will now be necessary. Confirm that they are happy to be lain horizontal before moving the chairback downwards. Ensure that the patient is comfortable and adjust the headrest as necessary. All new patients should have a full extra-oral examination prior to looking inside the mouth.

The extra-oral examination

First, observe the patient for any signs of obvious facial asymmetry.

Then examine the temporomandibular joints and associated structures. Place one finger on each mandibular condyle and ask the patient to slowly open the mouth wide and then close. Look for any deviation of the mandible on opening or closing. Feel and listen for any sounds from the joints such as clicking or crepitus. Check there is no tenderness in the joint regions. As well as the extent of opening, lateral movements of the mandible should be checked for any restrictions by asking the patient to open slightly and then move their jaw from side to side (fig. 2.4). Check the submandibular and cervical lymph nodes for any enlargement or tenderness.

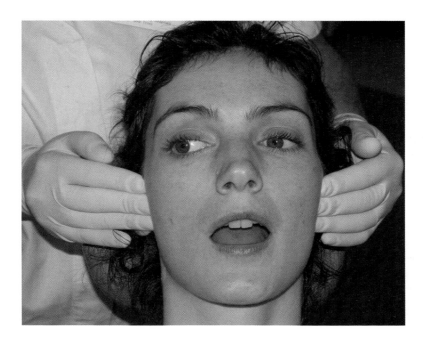

Figure 2.4 Palpating the TMJs.

The intra-oral examination

For an intra-oral examination, one needs a mirror, a straight probe, a Briault probe, a WHO periodontal probe and a pair of tweezers.

The soft tissues

Always look at the soft tissues first before examining the teeth. Develop a systematic approach so that you always examine the mouth in the same order – it will then become a routine.

Examine the lips, tongue, floor of the mouth, cheeks, hard and soft palate before looking initially at the general state of the gingivae. Note any unusual features in the patient records, with a simple drawing for clarification if necessary.

The teeth

Chart the teeth accurately, describing any restorations in terms of the surfaces of the teeth that they cover. This examination should primarily be visual using a mirror and an air syringe to dry the teeth (fig. 2.5). Always warn the patient that you are going to use the air syringe as it can be quite alarming for some patients, especially if they have sensitive teeth. The visual examination can be enhanced by placing cotton rolls in the upper buccal sulci to keep the cheeks out of the way.

A probe should only be used to clear any debris or plaque from the teeth or to confirm a visual finding e.g. a cavity. As well as a standard dental probe, a Briault probe is essential to examine more inaccessible areas.

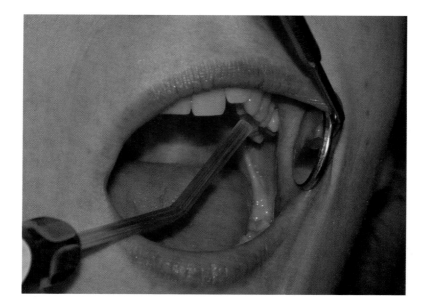

Figure 2.5 Using a mirror and 3-in-1.

The periodontal tissues

A basic periodontal examination (BPE) should be carried out using a WHO periodontal probe. This is a ball-ended probe with a black band 3.5–5.5 mm from the tip. In the BPE the mouth is divided into six sextants (UR8–UR4, UR3–UL3, UL4–UL8, LL8–LL4, LL3–LR3, LR4–LR8). A sextant must have at least two functioning teeth to be scored. Six sites are probed on each tooth, three on the buccal (mesial, distal and midpoint) and three on lingual or palatal (mesial, distal and midpoint). The probing force should ideally be 25 grams at each site.

Each sextant is graded from 0–4 using the following criteria:

0 No disease.
1 Gingival bleeding on probing but no pocketing, calculus or overhanging restorations.
2 Presence of supra- or subgingival calculus or plaque retention factors such as an overhanging restoration. No pockets of greater than 3 mm i.e. the black band on the WHO probe is still totally visible.
3 Pockets of 4–5 mm depth are present i.e. the black band on the probe is only partially visible.
4 Pockets of 6 mm or greater are present i.e. the black band on the probe is no longer visible.

The highest score in each sextant is recorded on a grid (fig. 2.6). A score of 3 or 4 in any sextant requires a more detailed periodontal assessment to assess the level of bone loss. A patient may have a score of 3 in only one sextant because of a particular problem at one site. A score of 3 in three or more sextants indicates a more generalised periodontal problem that needs to be investigated. Patients with a score of 4 in any sextant must always have a full periodontal assessment including plaque and bleeding scores, periodontal pocket charting, measurement of furcation involvement and tooth mobility assessment.

Plaque scores

The patient's oral hygiene can be assessed using a plaque scoring system. A disclosing solution is applied to all of the teeth so that the plaque can be easily visualised. Always remember to apply vaseline to the lips prior to applying the disclosing solution to prevent the solution staining the lips. Then, by

UR8–UR4	UR3–UL3	UL4–UL8
3	1	2
4	2	3
LR8–LR4	LR3–LL3	LL4–LL8

Figure 2.6 Basic periodontal examination (BPE) scoring grid.

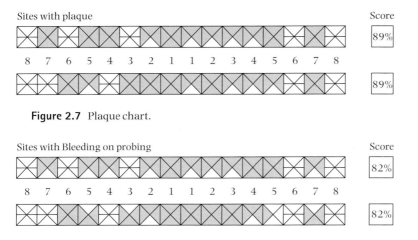

Sites with plaque   Score

8 7 6 5 4 3 2 1 1 2 3 4 5 6 7 8

89%

89%

Figure 2.7 Plaque chart.

Sites with Bleeding on probing   Score

8 7 6 5 4 3 2 1 1 2 3 4 5 6 7 8

82%

82%

Figure 2.8 Bleeding chart.

using a probe, the presence or absence of plaque is noted on four surfaces of each standing tooth – the mesial, buccal, distal and lingual/palatal surfaces. The results are plotted on a plaque scoring chart (fig. 2.7) and a percentage plaque score is calculated. This is the percentage of sites with plaque present out of the total number of sites tested.

A baseline plaque score percentage should be recorded at the beginning of treatment so that any changes can be monitored after oral hygiene instruction has been given. An improvement in oral hygiene may be an important factor in deciding whether to embark on complex restorative treatment.

Bleeding scores

Bleeding on probing the gingival sulcus is associated with gingival inflammation and is therefore an important indicator of disease. Gingival bleeding is recorded at four sites on each standing tooth – mesial, buccal, distal and lingual/palatal. A WHO periodontal probe is inserted to the base of the gingival sulcus at each site and moved gently along the tooth or root surface. After five seconds, the presence or absence of bleeding is noted and recorded on a chart (fig. 2.8). The bleeding score is the percentage of bleeding sites out of the total number of sites examined.

A baseline measurement of the bleeding score will give an indication of the level of gingival inflammation and, when taken with subsequent bleeding scores recorded during treatment, will show any improvements in the condition of the gingival tissues following periodontal therapy.

Periodontal pocket charting

A periodontal pocket is the distance in millimetres between the gingival margin and the base of the gingival sulcus and is measured with a graduated periodontal probe such a William's probe. In a healthy periodontium, the gingival sulcus is normally 1–2 mm in depth. Periodontal pocketing of greater than 3.5 mm is usually associated with alveolar bone loss but there can also be what is termed false pocketing, where gingival swelling and inflammation cause the gingival sulcus depth to be greater without any alveolar bone loss.

The probing pocket depths are recorded at six sites on each standing tooth – mesio-buccal, buccal, disto-buccal, disto-lingual or disto-palatal, lingual or palatal, mesio-lingual or mesio-palatal. The values are recorded on a chart (fig. 2.9) with the date of the examination clearly recorded.

Research has shown that probing pocket depths can vary according to the thickness of the probe used, the force and direction that the probe is inserted into the sulcus and also the level of inflammation present in the gingival tissues. The recommended probing force is 25 grams but this is difficult to apply

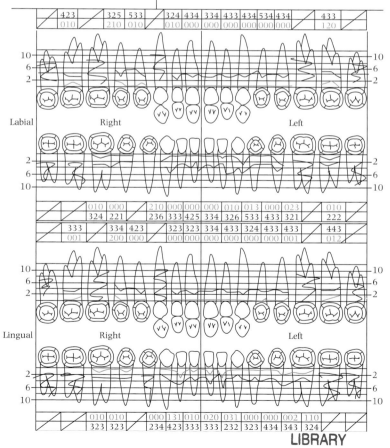

Figure 2.9 Pocket chart.

consistently unless one is using a pressure-sensitive probe with a predetermined force limit. One must therefore be aware of the limitations and accuracy of probing pocket depth measurements.

Probing pocket depths should be recorded prior to any periodontal therapy such as supra- and subgingival scaling or root planing so that any subsequent measurements can hopefully demonstrate an improvement.

Measurement of furcation involvement

If periodontal bone loss and gingival recession occurs in multi-rooted teeth, eventually the bifurcation or trifurcation area of the root will be exposed. This is significant because the furcation areas are usually inaccessible to normal plaque control methods and therefore disease in these areas is difficult to arrest. Therefore, the presence and level of furcation involvement must be recorded.

Furcation sites are classified as follows:

Level 1 – Horizontal loss of supporting tissues not exceeding 1/3 of the width of the tooth.

Level 2 – Horizontal loss of supporting tissues exceeding 1/3 of the width of the tooth, but not encompassing the total width of the furcation area.

Level 3 – Horizontal 'through and through' destruction of the supporting tissues in the furcation.

Mobility assessment

Progressive loss of alveolar bone will eventually lead to tooth mobility. Excessive tooth mobility can lead to pain and patient discomfort on eating. Tooth mobility can be classified as follows:

Level 1 – Movement of the tooth of 0.2–1 mm in a horizontal direction.

Level 2 – Movement of the tooth of greater than 1 mm in a horizontal direction.

Level 3 – Movement of the tooth in a vertical as well as a horizontal direction.

It must be remembered that abnormal tooth mobility can be caused by other factors such as abnormal occlusal load or trauma. These possible factors must be taken into account in your treatment planning.

Loss of attachment

If periodontal bone loss is accompanied by gingival recession, then there can be considerable loss of supporting tissues without there necessarily being any periodontal pocketing. Therefore some clinicians prefer to measure loss of attachment which is the distance in millimetres from the cement–enamel junction to the base of the gingival sulcus.

SPECIAL TESTS

Following the initial examination of the soft tissues, teeth and periodontal tissues, you must then decide if any special tests are needed. These could be one or more of the following:
- Radiographs
- Vitality testing
- Dietary analysis
- Percussion of the teeth
- Articulated study casts
- Diagnostic wax-up
- Photographs
- Tooth Wear Index

Radiographs

Since the patient is a new patient, it is unlikely that you have any previous radiographs unless the patient has brought copies of ones taken previously. There are well-established selection criteria for dental radiography. A useful radiograph is one whose result (positive or negative) will alter patient management. A significant number of radiographs do not fulfil this criterion and this unnecessary treatment increases costs as well as adding to patient irradiation.

Most fully or partially dentate patients will benefit from bitewing radiographs of each side of the mouth to show the crowns of the posterior teeth, crestal bone, any existing restorations and calculus deposits (fig. 2.10). These may then be supplemented with periapical radiographs of any teeth with signs or symptoms, as well as any teeth that are likely to need an indirect restoration (fig. 2.11).

Panoramic radiographs do not give a clear image of caries or apical pathology. They should only be used where the information cannot be gained through the use of intra-oral films. There is no justification for using panoramic radiography as a screening measure for new patients. Where possible, panoramic radiography should be restricted to the one side of the mouth where a problem exists, or, if one is examining for the presence of third molars, to the posterior regions only.

All radiographs should be mounted and a written report completed, preferably in consultation with a radiologist or suitable dental colleague.

Vitality testing

The vitality of a tooth means the integrity of the nerve supply within the pulpal complex. An intact nerve supply is reliant on an intact blood supply. Vitality can be tested by using a cold or hot stimulus or a small electric current through an electric pulp tester. The reliability of vitality tests can be questionable and

(a)

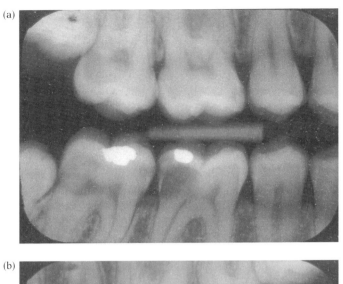

(b)

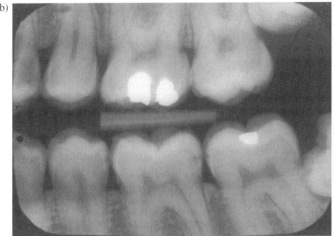

Figure 2.10 Left and right bitewing radiographs. Caries can be seen as follows: UR6 caries mesially into dentine; UR4 caries distally into dentine; LR7 caries mesially into dentine and caries occlusally distal to the occlusal amalgam; LR6 gross caries involving the distal pulp horn; UL4 caries distally well into dentine; LL5 caries distally in enamel only; LL6 caries distally into dentine; LL7 caries mesially in enamel only.

therefore the results of these tests should be assessed with any other clinical information gained.

The most common cold stimulus used is ethyl chloride. The tooth or teeth to be tested are isolated with dry cotton wool rolls. The ethyl chloride is sprayed on to a cotton pledget and this is then applied to each tooth in turn. The patient is asked whether they can feel the cold stimulus on the tooth. The time taken to react is noted – teeth with inflamed pulps may be hypersensitive

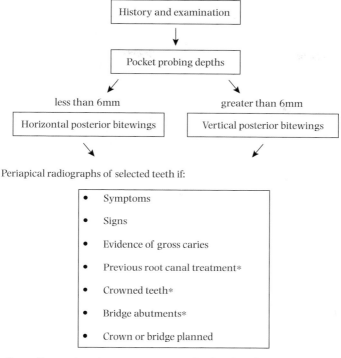

Periapical radiographs of selected teeth if:

- Symptoms
- Signs
- Evidence of gross caries
- Previous root canal treatment*
- Crowned teeth*
- Bridge abutments*
- Crown or bridge planned

*Depending on time since restoration completed and availability of previous radiographs.

Figure 2.11 Initial radiographic examination for a dentate or partially dentate patient.

to cold and the patient may react very suddenly. Using ethyl chloride is not a particularly reliable test in that a negative result does not automatically mean that the tooth is non-vital (fig. 2.12).

A hot stimulus is provided by heating a stick of gutta percha and then applying a small piece to the tooth on a flat plastic hand instrument. Gutta percha is quite adhesive so Vaseline should be applied to the teeth to prevent sticking.

Electric pulp testers have developed over the years. The older types had an earthing rod which the patient held and a pulse of current was then applied at each setting until the patient indicated that they could feel sensation. The modern types impart a continuous current at a consistent rate and have a digital readout which can then be recorded in the patient records. The advantage of the electric pulp tester is that it gives a numerical score which can be recorded and compared to previous or future scores to monitor vitality. The fact that it is an electric current needs to be carefully explained to the patient

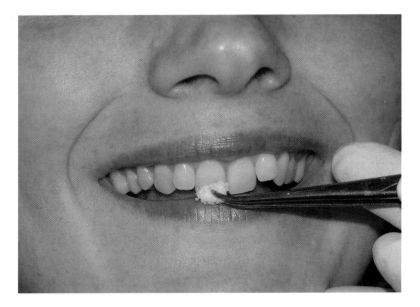

Figure 2.12 Using ethyl chloride.

so that they are not alarmed. Most pulp testers require the operator to have an ungloved hand to complete the electrical circuit.

Dietary analysis

Dietary analysis is an essential part of any treatment plan for a patient who is caries-active or who has pathology that may be diet-related e.g. tooth surface loss due to erosion. It is a record of all food and drink taken over a three-day period that should include one weekend day and should include any snacks or drinks taken between meals (see figs 9.3 and 9.15). The time that the food or drink was taken is recorded together with the quantity e.g. one cup of tea, one slice of toast.

It is always advisable to try to get the patient to complete the diet record throughout the day rather than trying to remember what has been consumed at the end of the day.

When the diet record is returned, it is analysed and advice given to the patient. The analysis looks first at the pattern of meals – does the patient have a structured diet in terms of three meals per day or is the pattern less defined? Then the number and frequency of sugar intakes is examined. Sugar intakes at meal times are less damaging than those in between meals. Frequent sugar intakes during the day e.g. sugar in tea or coffee, lower the oral pH and increase the chance of enamel demineralisation.

Diet advice to patients must be reasonable and achievable otherwise it will be ignored. Although there may be various risk factors identified in the diet record, it is preferable to start with one factor that can be changed e.g. cutting down the level of sugar in tea/coffee from two spoonfuls to one, or changing from sugar to an artificial sweetener. Once progress has been achieved with one factor, then another area of concern can be raised. Diet advice should always be couched as help for the patient in trying to overcome a present problem as well as preventing future problems.

Percussion of the teeth

Percussion of the teeth can be a useful diagnostic test when the patient has symptoms but cannot identify precisely where the problem is coming from. If a patient has pain, it is preferable to initially just use finger pressure on the teeth involved in case they are very periostitic. If this does not produce symptoms, then the teeth can be percussed with the end of a mouth mirror or probe. This can be done on the occlusal surface down the long axis of the tooth, or from the buccal side to test for pain on lateral movement (fig. 2.13). Where a cracked cusp is suspected, individual tooth cusps can be percussed in turn to examine for sensitivity.

Articulated study casts

Study casts are an invaluable aid particularly in cases where crowns, bridgework or partial dentures are contemplated. Ideally these should be mounted

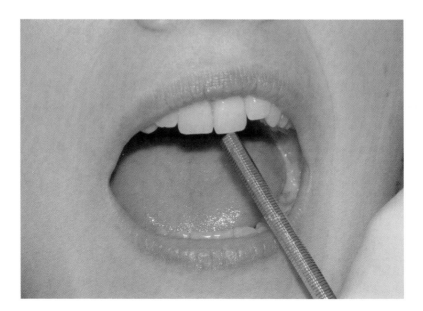

Figure 2.13 A percussion test.

on a semi-adjustable articulator by means of a facebow transfer, but in simple cases it may be adequate to have models set up on an average value articulator in the first instance.

Study casts must be surveyed prior to partial denture design so that all the preparatory treatment can be planned prior to the taking of the working impressions. This may be simple measures such as the cutting of rest seats, or it may be modification of the abutment teeth by placing crowns or the addition of composite resin to increase the level of undercut present.

Diagnostic wax-up

If a major change is to be made to the shape or position of the teeth, then it is sometimes useful to ask your technician to construct a diagnostic wax-up of what the teeth might look like when finished. If it is proposed to close an upper central diastema, for example, with veneers or crowns, a wax-up can show both the patient and the operator the final width and shape of the teeth. If a bridge is proposed and there has been abnormal alveolar bone loss in the pontic area, a diagnostic wax-up will show the potential length and width of the pontics in relation to the retainers and the other teeth. If pontics have to be very long, they can look artificial and unnatural which might then be an indicator to use a removable partial denture with a gingival flange rather than a fixed bridge.

Another use for the diagnostic wax-up model is in the construction of a suck-down splint to construct temporary restorations. When the study model has been waxed up, it is then duplicated in stone and used as a base for a vacuum-formed suck-down splint. The advantages of this in temporisation are mainly in multi-unit crown and bridgework where individual temporary restorations are not possible. In other cases where restorations have fractured or where the vertical dimensions are being increased, the original teeth or restorations are not applicable as guides to the temporary restorations. This is where a splint made from a waxed-up model can be invaluable. It also has the advantage that it can be reused time and again which can be very useful in emergency situations where temporary restorations have been lost or damaged.

Photography

Pre- and post-operative photographs are an invaluable aid in treatment planning. Five photographs are normally taken to show the teeth and supporting tissues. These are anterior, left and right lateral views with the teeth in occlusion and occlusal mirror views of the upper and lower arches. Photographs can show patients what has been achieved during the treatment and can also be used to demonstrate to other patients what could be achieved in their cases if treatment of a similar type were proposed.

As well as conventional SLR and digital cameras, there are also many intra-oral camera systems available today. These can be very useful in treatment planning to show patients the extent of intra-oral problems of which they may not be aware e.g. a fractured restoration.

The computer software that comes with these systems can also be used to manipulate images on the screen to show patients how the appearance of their teeth can be altered e.g. closing a diastema, correcting rotations, changing the colour of the teeth. Seeing a change to a photographic image of their own teeth will be much more relevant to the patient than looking at a plaster model or a diagnostic wax-up. The challenge to the operator is then to ensure that the final results are as good as the predicted result.

Tooth Wear Index

Non-carious tooth tissue loss is an increasing problem as life expectancy increases and patients retain their teeth for longer. As it will normally be progressive, it is important to monitor the situation carefully. Sequential study models and photographs can be used as can the Tooth Wear Index proposed by Smith and Knight in 1984. This index records a score for each unrestored surface of each standing tooth (fig. 2.14). What is defined as pathological will depend on the age of the patient and acceptable levels for the upper cervical surfaces have been set for each age group (fig. 2.15).

Score*	Surface	Criterion
0	B/L/O/I C	No loss of enamel surface characteristics No change of contour
1	B/L/O/I C	Loss of enamel surface characteristics Minimal loss of contour
2	B/L/O I C	Loss of enamel exposing dentine for less than one-third of the surface Loss of enamel just exposing dentine Defect less than 1 mm deep
3	B/L/O I C	Loss of enamel exposing dentine for more than one-third of the surface Loss of enamel and substantial loss of dentine, but not exposing pulp or secondary dentine Defect 1–2 mm deep
4	B/L/O I C	Complete loss of enamel, or pulp exposure, or exposure of secondary dentine Pulp exposure or exposure of secondary dentine Defect of more than 2 mm deep, or pulp exposure, or exposure of secondary dentine

*In case of doubt a lower score is given**
B = buccal or labial; L = lingual or palatal; O = occlusal; I = incisal; C = cervical

Figure 2.14 Classification of the Tooth Wear Index (Smith and Knight 1984).

Age	UR8	UR7	UR6	UR5	UR4	UR3	UR2	UR1	UL1	UL2	UL3	UL4	UL5	UL6	UL7	UL8
<25	0	0	0	1	1	1	0	0	0	0	1	1	1	0	0	0
26–35	1	1	1	1	1	1	1	1	1	1	1	1	1	1	1	1
36–45	1	1	1	2	2	2	1	1	1	1	2	2	2	1	1	1
46–55	1	1	1	2	2	2	2	2	2	2	2	2	2	1	1	1
56–65	1	1	1	2	2	2	2	2	2	2	2	2	2	1	1	1
>65	1	1	1	2	2	2	2	2	2	2	2	2	2	1	1	1

Figure 2.15 Acceptable levels of toothwear of the upper cervical surfaces (Smith and Knight 1984).

CONCLUSION

Once all the information has been collected, the clinician needs to consider all the possible options before sitting down with the patient to discuss the best treatment for that patient at that moment in time.

In the next chapter we will discuss patient management.

3 Patient management

INTRODUCTION

In this chapter, we will look at the common medical problems of patients in general dental practice and the relevance of those problems to the treatment of the patient. We will then look at the treatment of anxious patients and give practical advice on their management.

COMMON MEDICAL PROBLEMS

With the demographic shift in the population, the size of the elderly population is increasing. This increase in life expectancy is often the result of improved treatment of previously debilitating or fatal diseases. As a consequence, many patients are taking one or more pharmaceutical drugs, which may be of relevance in relation to dental treatment. As many more elderly patients are retaining their teeth this is an increasing problem which dentists must address.

Cardiovascular problems

The most common cardiovascular disorders that dentists will meet in their patients are *hypertension* and *ischaemic coronary heart disease.*

Hypertension may be either primary in nature or secondary to other medical problems such as renal, endocrine or cerebral disorders. As well as drug therapy, it is treated by a number of non-pharmacological methods. Patients are advised to cease smoking, reduce their salt and alcohol intake, take more exercise and lose weight, if that is applicable. Antihypertensive drugs such as beta blockers, angiotensin-converting enzyme inhibitors or calcium-channel blockers are often used in combination with a diuretic, usually from the thiazide group.

Ischaemic coronary heart disease is a progressive reduction in coronary blood flow due to narrowing of the coronary vessels. Hypertension is a major contributory factor. If untreated, coronary heart disease can lead to either angina or myocardial infarction. Both of these are due to ischaemia but angina is usually precipitated by exertion whereas a myocardial infarction may start with little or no warning. Angina is treated with glyceryl trinitrate together with antihypertensive drugs. In addition aspirin, which thins the blood through its antiplatelet activity, is often prescribed.

Patients with cardiovascular disease need careful management but there is no reason why they cannot be treated in general dental practice. There is some debate about whether adrenaline-containing local anaesthetics should be used in these patients in case some anaesthetic gets into the bloodstream and causes generalised systemic effects. If an aspirating syringe is used, the chances of an intravascular injection are reduced. What is much more likely to be significant is an increase in the endogenous level of adrenaline if the patient is in pain or is anxious. Therefore, treatment should be well planned with short appointments if possible, preferably in the morning. Local anaesthesia must be effective, with topical local anaesthesia being used to make the injections as painless as possible.

Antibiotic prophylaxis

Antibiotics are sometimes given prophylactically before treatment to prevent post-operative complications or infection. In general dental practice, the most common reason for antibiotic prophylaxis is in the prevention of infective endocarditis (IE). The link between dental treatment and infective endocarditis is increasingly being questioned but it is accepted that if the patient is at risk and is undergoing a procedure that is likely to induce a significant bacteraemia, antibiotic prophylaxis should be administered. Antibiotics have been massively overused by the medical and dental professions and this has resulted in the development of many organisms which are now resistant to many common antibiotics. We must therefore be careful to ensure that any antibiotics prescribed are definitely indicated.

The guidelines to follow are:

- *Identify whether the patient is at risk of contracting IE.* Patients *at high risk* are those with a prosthetic heart valve or those who have previously had endocarditis. Patients also *at risk but at a lower level* are those with congenital heart disease, rheumatic or other valvular heart disease and surgically constructed systemic pulmonary shunts. Patients *not at risk* include those who have had a myocardial infarction, coronary bypass surgery, or have a pacemaker in place. Many patients give a history of having a heart murmur. These have often been discovered during a routine examination and are symptomless. Unless the patient has been examined by a cardiologist and has been shown to have valvular damage, the risk of contracting IE is negligible. These patients do not need antibiotic prophylaxis. The peak incidence of IE is in the sixth and seventh decades of life, so the elderly are at more risk than younger patients.
- *Decide which treatments need prophylactic antibiotics.* Prophylaxis is needed where the treatment is likely to cause a significant bacteraemia. The keyword here is *significant*, as almost all oral activities including eating and toothbrushing have been shown to cause a bacteraemia at some level. The current recommendations are that prophylaxis is mandatory for extractions, supra- and subgingival scaling, periodontal surgery, reimplantation of avulsed teeth and incision and drainage of infected tissue.
- *Give the correct antibiotic at the correct time.* The recommended regimes for antibiotic prophylaxis are documented in the *Dental Practitioner's Formulary.* Oral antibiotics should be given one hour prior to the procedure, intravenous antibiotics may be given just before the procedure.

Haematological disorders and anticoagulated patients

Dentists may occasionally come across patients who have a congenital coagulation disorder such as haemophilia. However, they are much more likely to see patients with an acquired coagulation defect, principally patients who are on anticoagulant therapy such as warfarin. All patients who are on warfarin will have regular blood tests, the results of which are recorded in a distinctive yellow booklet. The results record the International Normalised Ratio (INR) which is the ratio of the patient's clotting time to the normal clotting time. The INR is usually maintained at between 2.5 and 3.5 for most patients, 3.5–4.5 for patients at higher risk.

The advice for the treatment of anticoagulated patients who require an extraction or other procedure that might cause bleeding, has recently changed. Previously, the anticoagulant dose was withdrawn for 48 hours to allow the warfarin to clear the system and then the INR was rechecked. Now the advice is that patients with an INR of less than 4.0 can have extractions or other procedures without their anticoagulant dose being reduced. This change of policy is based on the hazards to the patient of altering the anti-coagulant dose; also, research that has shown that anticoagulated patients who have extractions do not bleed excessively, provided appropriate local measures are taken. These are:

- The extraction(s) should be as atraumatic as possible.
- A local anaesthetic using a vasoconstrictor should be administered by infiltration or intraligamentary injection wherever practical.
- After extraction, sockets should be gently packed with an absorbable haemostatic dressing e.g. oxidised cellulose (Surgicel®) or collagen sponge (Haemocollagen®), then carefully sutured. Pressure should be applied by using a gauze pad that the patient bites down on for 15–30 minutes.
- Clear post-operative instructions must be given on measures to be taken if bleeding recommences and emergency contact telephone numbers must be issued.

The patient's general medical practitioner or the haematologist in charge of the anticoagulation should *always* be approached for advice prior to any extractions or procedure likely to induce significant bleeding.

Respiratory disorders

The incidence of asthma has increased greatly over the past twenty years and dentists will regularly encounter patients who are using various inhalers to control this disease. Some of these may contain corticosteroids and the possibility of adrenal suppression must be considered for patients who have been using steroids over long periods of time.

Treatment under general anaesthesia is to be avoided where possible for patients with respiratory disorders but treatment under local anaesthesia poses few problems. Anxiety may occasionally precipitate asthmatic attacks and it is therefore important to reduce the fear of dental treatment by gentle handling and reassurance.

Patients with chronic respiratory disorders may have problems lying horizontal in the dental chair and may need treatment in a semi-prone position.

Gastrointestinal disorders

Patients with gastrointestinal disorders may have problems taking medication that a dentist may prescribe such as antibiotics or analgesics.

Gastric reflux is a cause of non-carious tooth tissue loss.

Liver disease

Liver disease is important in treatment planning because of possible bleeding tendencies and impaired drug detoxification.

Diabetes

Patients with diabetes are more prone to periodontal disease and tend to heal more slowly after extractions or minor oral surgery.

MANAGING THE ANXIOUS PATIENT

Assessment of anxiety

Both qualitative and quantitative measures of dental anxiety can be made.

The qualitative measures can be made by observation. The patient may be shaking, sweating and be unwilling or uncertain about sitting in the dental chair. Patients who are nervous often talk incessantly, others avoid eye contact. We can also gain important information through the dental history that the patient gives. There may have been a previous bad dental experience which has affected the patient's confidence in the dentist.

Dental anxiety can be measured quantitatively using a questionnaire. There are many dental anxiety questionnaires but the quickest and simplest is the Modified Dental Anxiety Scale (MDAS). This questionnaire (fig. 2.2) has five questions relating to different aspects of dental treatment including scaling, drilling and local anaesthetic injections. The range of scores is from 5 to 25. The average score is around 11; those with high anxiety score 20+.

Prevention of anxiety

A lot of patient anxiety follows a bad dental experience. It can take only one distressing episode to affect a patient's attitude for many years. It is therefore particularly important to try to prevent any experience that may colour a patient's attitude to dentistry in the future. There are two situations that tend to recur as bad experiences. The first is where a procedure becomes unexpectedly more complex e.g. a forceps extraction turning into a surgical extraction, and the second is where a patient feels pain during a procedure. Therefore, the key elements are good planning and good pain control.

Planning for anxious patients

As we have emphasised before, good communication skills are vital in treatment planning. This is especially so with anxious patients. Many patients, especially when they are anxious, do not remember all that they have been told during dental visits. To take account of this, there are some simple guidelines that can be followed:

- Ensure that the information that you are giving is in plain, simple, jargon-free language. Clarify your message by asking the patient if they have understood and if they have any questions.
- Reinforce your message by repeating it.

- Give your patient control over the procedure by the use of stop signals e.g. raising the hand.
- Tell the patient what is going to happen as the procedure progresses. Most patients are happiest when they know what is going to happen next, although a few may request no details at all – 'Just get on with it, I don't want to know'.
- Ensure that the patient knows what is to happen at the next visit. If the patient feels the next procedure may be difficult for them, they can prepare in advance and may bring someone with them for support.

Pain control

Good pain control is achieved through effective local anaesthesia which should be given as painlessly as possible. This is achieved by the use of topical local anaesthetic cream or spray so that the patient is less likely to feel the prick of the needle. Once through the mucosa, a slow injection rate is used as the needle is passed to the optimum point. The needle should follow the local anaesthetic solution through the tissues so that an *anaesthetic pathway* is produced. Warming the local anaesthetic solution to near body temperature will also make the patient less aware of the injection.

Some local anaesthetic injections will take more time to work than others. Intraosseous anaesthesia can give almost instantaneous results whereas an inferior dental block may take 10–15 minutes to be effective. Whatever type of injection you have given, always check your anaesthesia before proceeding. Check for soft tissue anaesthesia in the area supplied by the nerve you have blocked, and then ask the patient if they are happy for you to proceed. The trust between you and the patient will be lost if you try to start before the patient is numb.

Anxious patients often have a low pain threshold. If they use a stop signal to halt the procedure, you *must* respond to their concerns. If they are feeling pain, additional local anaesthesic should be administered. If you are happy that your primary injection i.e. infiltration or block, is effective, then the use of intraligamentary or intraosseous anaesthesia is indicated. The mere fact that you have stopped and are trying to gain more effective anaesthesia is reassuring to the patient and will reinforce the trust between you.

4 Reaching a diagnosis

What is diagnosis? Diagnosis is a Greek-derived word meaning decision. Diagnosis is not an end in itself; it is a mental resting place for prognostic considerations and therapeutic decisions.

Ekstrand *et al.* 2001

INTRODUCTION

Now you have gathered all the relevant information, you can work out a diagnosis. This is critical to the success of the treatment. Only by formulating a diagnosis can you plan treatment. If you have not correctly diagnosed the case, the treatment you provide may be ineffective or unsuccessful.

Once you have completed your initial history and examination, you will often have an idea of what the diagnosis will be. This expertise will come with experience to a certain extent in that the more often you hear a certain history or list of symptoms or the more you see a problem, the more likely you are to recognise the cause; thus common dental pathology such as caries or periodontal disease is usually easy to diagnose with a careful clinical examination supplemented by appropriate special tests. However, the aetiology of the disease process that you have diagnosed may be more difficult to define.

A common example of this is toothwear which may be due to erosion, attrition, abrasion, abfraction or a combination of any of these.

COMMON DIAGNOSES

Periodontal diseases

Gingivitis

The diagnosis of plaque-induced gingivitis is usually made from the visual appearance. The gingivae will be red and swollen, with a loss of stippling. Careful probing should be used to assess active bleeding sites and to confirm the absence of bone loss. Probing may also be used to assess plaque traps, such as subgingival calculus deposits and the presence of ledges on restorations. Visual examination, the use of a probe and disclosing solution will identify the plaque deposits that cause the disease process. Radiographic examination is not indicated for the diagnosis of gingivitis.

Chronic periodontitis

This disease is characterised by the loss of attachment, apical migration of the junctional epithelium and bone loss. On visual examination you should look for signs of gingivitis, supragingival and subgingival calculus deposits, drifting and recession (fig. 4.1). Probing should be used to assess pocket depth, furcation involvement and bleeding from the base of the pocket, the latter being an indicator for active disease. Probing may also reveal suppuration, furcation involvement, ledges on restorations and subgingival calculus deposits. Probe and/or mirror handles should be used to assess tooth mobility. Radiographs, such as vertical bitewings, may be used to confirm bone loss and sequential pocket charts may be used to assess disease progression.

Dental caries

Diagnosis of dental caries involves detecting a lesion and making an assessment of the lesion activity. The lesion may be progressing rapidly or

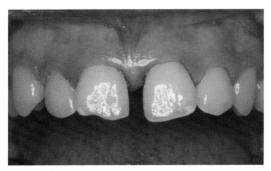

Figure 4.1 Periodontal disease.

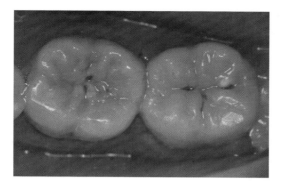

Figure 4.2 Occlusal caries.

slowly or may already be arrested. If carious lesions can be diagnosed in their early stages, the dynamic balance may be tipped in favour of repair by modifying the diet and the use of fluorides.

Caries may be detected by direct visual examination (fig. 4.2). You need to look at the colour of the enamel, shadows within dentine, the shape and texture of the lesion and whether it is cavitated. The colour of the carious dentine, whether occlusal or root caries, is no longer considered to be an indicator of disease activity. The important indicators of active lesions are softness and wetness of the dentine. It is important to remove all plaque and air-dry the tooth. Air-drying replaces water in the porous demineralised enamel with air and the lesion becomes more obvious owing to the difference in refractive indices of air and enamel. The clinical appearance of occlusal caries can be related to the lesion's activity, the level of infection in dentine and the histopathology by using a ranked scoring system (see Table 4.1).

Supplementary diagnostic techniques may also be used. The bitewing radiograph is a very valuable adjunct, especially for approximal caries and may also be used for recurrent, root and occlusal caries. Magnification will improve the diagnostic yield from conventional film radiographs. Other techniques include fibre optic transillumination, electrical conductance, lasers and salivary flow and bacterial activity tests.

Failed restorations

The reason given most often for the failure of restorations is dental caries, but there are many other reasons why restorations are considered to have failed. These may include other biological problems such as gingival recession around restoration margins or abrasion resulting in wear of the dental material as well as tooth tissue. Mechanical failure of restorations through fracture, wear or marginal breakdown is not uncommon. Iatrogenic causes, such as ledges and deficiencies, may mean that restorations are removed and replaced. Patients may wish restorations replaced because of poor appearance,

Table 4.1 Occlusal caries lesion appearances, activity, histopathology and level of infection (from Ekstrand *et al.* 2001).

Score	Clinical appearance	Activity	Histopathology	Level of infection
0	No, or slight change in enamel translucency after prolonged air-drying (>5s)	Probably none	No enamel demineralisation or a narrow surface zone of opacity (edge phenomenon)	0
1	Opacity (white) hardly visible on the wet surface but distinctly visible after air-drying	Active	Enamel demineralisation limited to the outer 50% of the enamel layer	0
1a	Opacity (brown) hardly visible on the wet surface but distinctly visible after air-drying	Arrested		0
2	Opacity (white) distinctly visible without air-drying	Active	Demineralisation involving 50% of the enamel and up to 1/3 of the dentine	+
2a	Opacity (brown) distinctly visible without air-drying	Arrested		+
3	Localised enamel break-down in opaque or discoloured enamel and/or greyish discolouration from the underlying dentine	Active	Demineralisation involving the middle 1/3 of the dentine	++
4	Cavitation in opaque or discoloured enamel exposing the dentine	Active	Demineralisation involving the inner 1/3 of the dentine	++++

perhaps because of changes in the colour of tooth-coloured restorations over time through stain acquisition or degeneration of the restorative material. Patients may also wish metal restorations replaced with tooth-coloured restorations for appearance, health or environmental concerns. Inappropriate contour such as poor emergence profile of crowns or positive and negative ledges on direct restorations can be another reason for replacing the restoration as such defects can contribute to gingival and periodontal problems. Fracture or wear of the restorative material, for example acrylic teeth on dentures, can also result in problems and the need for the replacement or repair of the restoration. Occlusal problems caused by wear or fracture or initial poor planning is another cause of failure. The diagnosis of such problems requires careful history taking, clinical examination and the use of appropriate special investigations if the same errors are not to be repeated.

Toothwear

The diagnosis of toothwear is made on the basis of the clinical examination, supplemented by the medical, social and clinical histories. Patients who grind their teeth may have tongue scalloping and hyperkeratosis (a white line) at the occlusal level on the buccal mucosa. There will be a change in the appearance of the teeth; the crowns may be shorter than normal, cupping of the occlusal surfaces and incisal edges may be noted, dentine may be exposed, enamel may be thinner and restorations may be worn or proud of the surrounding tooth tissue. Patients may complain of pain or sensitivity owing to the exposed dentine or of facial muscle pain from parafunction. You may also notice a loss of occlusal vertical dimension. There are different patterns of toothwear associated with the various aetiologies, however it should be remembered that toothwear is often multifactorial, especially in the older patient.

Table 4.2 Classification of toothwear.

Type	Cause	Clinical pattern
Erosion (see fig. 4.3)	Chemical process in which tooth tissue is removed in the absence of plaque. Acid may be extrinsic (dietary) or intrinsic (stomach acid).	Often seen on palatal surfaces of upper anterior teeth and/or occlusal surfaces of posterior teeth. Surfaces appear smooth and shiny. Existing restorations may be proud of the tooth tissue.
Abrasion (see fig. 4.4)	External agents such as toothbrushes abrade tooth substance.	Usually seen at the buccal cervical margins of the upper teeth when the cause is vigorous toothbrushing.
Attrition (see fig. 4.5)	Tooth to tooth contact resulting in wear.	Seen on occlusal surfaces and incisal edges that are in contact with the opposing teeth in function or parafunction (bruxism).
Abfraction	Cusp flexure from loading causes stress at the cervical margin.	Wedge-shaped lesions at the cervical margins.

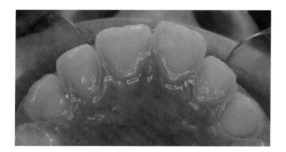

Figure 4.3 Erosion.

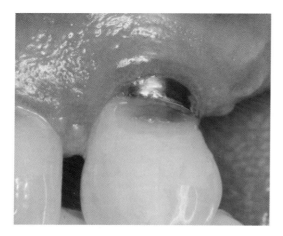

Figure 4.4 Abrasion.

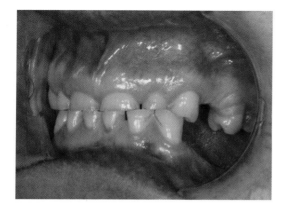

Figure 4.5 Attrition.

Dental trauma

The diagnosis of recent trauma will be based mainly on the history and clinical appearance. Radiographs may be required to assess for root fracture, which can be difficult to see initially. Parallax views may be required (remember the SLOB rule – same lingual, opposite buccal – i.e. if the object moves in the same direction as the x-ray tube then it is lingually placed). Vitality tests are of little diagnostic value at this stage but should be recorded to give baseline values. Trauma that has occurred in the past can present many years later as discolouration or pulpal/periapical problems, and can be more difficult to manage owing to the amount of reparative dentine that has been laid down.

Dentine hypersensitivity

The clinical history of dentine hypersensitivity is usually one of sharp pain in areas of exposed dentine and is elicited in response to external stimuli such as cold air, food or drinks. Clinical examination may reveal exposed root surfaces, a lost restoration or areas of worn tooth substance. Testing with an air blast, thermal stimuli or probing may be completed to confirm the diagnosis. The presence of dentine hypersensitivity is also taken as a sign that the toothwear process is ongoing.

Pulpal/periapical problems

The diagnosis of dental pain can be difficult, particularly if your patient does not give a clear history. There are several specific questions that you should ask in order to come to your diagnosis. They are:
- How intense is the pain? Is it constant and throbbing? Or short and sharp?
- Does it keep you awake at night?
- Can you eat on that side of your mouth?
- Is it worse when you eat or drink something hot or cold?
- Do painkillers help?

Having asked these questions you can start to come to a diagnosis, aided by careful clinical examination and special investigations such as vitality tests,

Table 4.3 Dental pain diagnosis

Symptoms							Diagnosis
Intense pain	Sleep disturbed	Painful to bite	Constant throbbing	Worse with hot	Short/sharp with cold	Painkillers help	
✗	✗	✗	✗	✗	✓	✓	Reversible pulpitis
✗	✓	✓	✓	✓	✗	✗	Irreversible pulpitis
✓	✓	✓	✓/✗	✗	✗	✗	Apical periodontitis

percussion and possibly radiographs, although the latter may be used more for the decision about treatment rather than actual diagnosis. Radiographs will certainly confirm the presence of long-standing periapical disease but will be of limited diagnostic value for new, acute problems. Instead, they are used to aid decisions about whether a tooth is restorable, whether it can be root-filled or the difficulty of extraction.

Cracked tooth

A cracked tooth can be difficult to diagnose. There may be clues in the mouth, such as the presence of very large direct restorations, visible cracks in the tooth or multiple wear facets, however, more often there are no such obvious signs. The classic symptom of a cracked tooth is sharp pain on release of a bit-ing force. Diagnostic techniques involve tapping the cusps of the suspected teeth from different directions, getting the patient to bite on a cotton wool roll or on a specially designed rubber stick known as a 'tooth slooth'. Careful examination of the tooth for cracks and probing around restoration margins may help. Sometimes on removal of a restoration in a suspected tooth, the cracked cusp will fly off, confirming the diagnosis.

Discoloured teeth

Discolouration of teeth is usually defined as intrinsic or extrinsic. Extrinsic discolouration may be caused by food stains such as tea, coffee, red wine and spices or by medications such as chlorhexidine mouthwash. Children often collect plaque that includes chromogenic bacteria and this is another cause of extrinsic staining. Extrinsic staining is recognised by the fact that it can be removed by prophylaxis paste or pumice and water in a rubber cup in a rotary instrument.

The common causes of intrinsic discolouration of vital teeth are tetra-cycline, fluorosis, and age. Tetracycline forms grey, brown and yellow pigmented fluorescent bands within developing teeth as a result of binding with the calcium in hydroxyapatite (the lower incisors in fig. 6.6). The severity of the pigmentation depends on three factors: the time and duration of administration, the type of tetracycline administered and the dosage. Fluoro-sis is caused by excessive concentrations of fluoride during enamel calcifica-tion. The high concentration of fluoride is believed to cause a metabolic alteration in the ameloblasts, resulting in a defective matrix and improper calcification. This is seen as brown and white mottling of the teeth (fig. 6.5a). The discolouration of teeth with age is thought to relate to a combination of extrinsic stains and physiological changes such as reparative dentine and tooth wear.

Discolouration can also occur in non-vital teeth and is commonly the result of trauma to upper incisors or poorly completed root canal treatment. As a result of trauma, or pulpal remains being incompletely extirpated from the pulp chamber, blood products from the pulp enter the dentine, resulting in a grey discolouration of the dentine (fig. 6.4a).

DENTURE PROBLEMS

Denture problems may divided into three main groups:
- Discomfort
- Looseness
- Problems of adaptation.

In order to work out what is causing the problem a careful history is required, followed by clinical examination of the facial profile, lip support, speech, the edentulous saddles/ridges and any remaining teeth. The following aspects of the dentures should be examined: occlusal vertical dimension, appearance, occlusion and articulation, extensions, tooth position, shape of the polished surfaces, stability and retention.

Discomfort

One of the causes of discomfort relates to the fitting surface of the denture which may be over- or underextended owing to impression errors or because of laboratory errors. The polished and occlusal surfaces of dentures are another source of denture pain and this will mainly be caused by incorrect occlusal registration or tooth positioning. Factors not relating to the dentures, such as xerostomia and burning mouth, can also present as denture discomfort.

Looseness

Dentures become loose when the displacing forces are greater than the retaining forces. Factors that increase the displacing forces include over-extended dentures, poor adaptation to the supporting tissues, incorrect tooth positioning, occlusal errors and anatomical problems such as a flabby or fibrous ridge, a large fraenum and bony prominences.

Problems of adaptation

Patients may not adapt to denture-wearing because of any of the problems mentioned above, but they may also have concerns about the function or the appearance of their new prosthesis. Some patients will take longer to develop denture-wearing skills than others and additional encouragement may be required.

5 Decision-making

INTRODUCTION

Once we have completed our clinical investigations and made a diagnosis we can then start to make decisions about providing the most appropriate care for our patients. There are many influences on our decisions. We know that for the same clinical finding, different treatments are provided for individual patients. This is not necessarily wrong; there are many factors that can and should influence treatment planning. A clinical consultation is not simply a matter of applying the available dental evidence to a given patient. Clinical judgement is a very important part of the decision-making process and should be integrated with the available evidence base in dentistry to provide the most appropriate care for our patients. The factors that should be taken into account in the planning of dental care do not relate solely to the clinical conditions with which the patient presents; many other factors are involved and this is why judgement is important. You have to be able to take account of patient factors – such as medical history – and dentist factors – such as your knowledge and skill. We can use the available evidence base in dentistry to inform our decisions but this is very limited in many areas. Clinical judgement is an extremely important part of the decision-making process.

WHAT IS INVOLVED IN MAKING DECISIONS ABOUT TREATMENT?

> No sensible decision can be made any longer without taking into account not only the world as it is, but the world as it will be . . .
>
> Isaac Asimov 1920–92

The first stage is to collect as much information from the patient as you can. With this information, whether it be the patient's concerns or clinical findings, you can then decide which special tests or investigations to carry out. Ideally, by this stage you will have found out what your patient's perception of his/her dental problem(s) is. Your patient may also have views on what they want done about their problem. Many patients acquire dental knowledge from the Internet and other sources and may have quite firm ideas about their management. You should also have established this, detected any disease and found out the causes of the disease in your patient. It should then be possible to make a diagnosis. The next stage is to consider all the treatment options: what is possible, the advantages and disadvantages of each option and the risks involved. It is important to take into account all the influences on care, such as medical and social history. Preferably you should discuss all the options with your patients in a clear and logical fashion. These options must be presented to the patient in a form they can understand and it is your responsibility to assess this. You should now be in a position to make a judgement on the best care for your patient and know either how to provide or how to obtain that care for your patient (fig. 5.1).

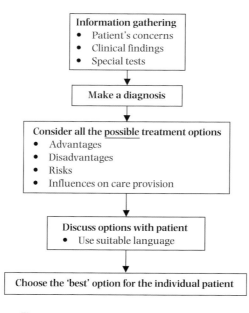

Figure 5.1 Treatment decisions flow chart.

WHAT FACTORS INFLUENCE DECISIONS ABOUT CARE?

Making decisions about treatment and planning care are complex processes that are influenced by many factors. These include those relating to the patient and the dentist, their interrelationship and factors relating to the clinical treatment options.

> The distribution of tooth extraction reflects not only the prevalence of underlying pathologies but also a complex combination of patients' and dentists' attitudes.
>
> Kay and Blinkhorn 1987

Patient factors

You will have found out many of these in your history taking. It is essential to use the answers that the patient gives you to inform the decision-making process.

First of all, you should find out whether your patient has any concerns about their dental health and what your patient wants and expects from treatment. This can be difficult as the patient may not know and will often say that no one has ever asked them. Of course, they may want different things from their dental care than you consider appropriate and it is important to establish this before treatment starts. They may have unrealistic expectations of what is achievable in terms of possible treatment options. For example, there is a general increase in patients' expectations of tooth longevity. They may have very strong ideas about the type of treatment they want. Conversely the patient may not want to be involved in the decision making process and may want you to make the decisions for them as they may feel that you know best.

The value an individual patient places on his/her teeth will affect the care that is provided. Any benefits that the patient may gain from dental treatment, such as improved appearance or the knowledge that there is no active disease present, must be worth the expenditure to them. Expenditure does not just mean financial cost but also the time spent, the anxiety associated with treatment or the difficulties in accessing care. Different dentists approach care in different ways and this can be confusing for the patient. Therefore it is important to have a diagnosis and to be able to explain the various treatment options to patients in terms that they can understand. People have differing attitudes towards risk. Some patients may be willing to try a treatment with limited longevity whereas others may want a less 'risky' option. This attitude towards risk can have a large effect on treatment planning. There are certain dental procedures that your patient may have strong feelings or concerns about. One common current concern is the use of dental amalgam as a restorative material. It is therefore essential to have a sound knowledge of such issues so that you can discuss them with your patients.

AMALGAM AND ILL HEALTH

Dental amalgam has been in use since the nineteenth century. Mercury is toxic but there is no credible scientific evidence to suggest that the minute amount of mercury released from dental amalgam restorations contributes to disease or has any toxicological effects in humans. True amalgam allergy is extremely rare. A number of investigations specifically related to the health problems associated with dental amalgam have been carried out. These studies have shown no link between amalgam and such complaints as headache and fatigue or between amalgam and cancer. It has also been shown that no symptoms among dental staff and their children can be related to the use of dental amalgam, assuming that correct hygiene measures are employed. Some studies have found other organic causes for the patients' complaints and this possibility should not be overlooked. Anaemia and other blood dyscrasias can also cause lethargy and headache.

The social history you obtained will impact on care. If the patient works shifts or works offshore or lives a long distance from the surgery then this can affect their attendance pattern and may limit the treatment options. Certain occupations or hobbies may also influence the type of care that you provide. Musicians may have specific requirements in terms of function and appearance. Habits may also limit treatment options: smoking may be a contraindication for implant treatment and it may also influence periodontal therapy. A high sugar intake in the diet may preclude complex restorative care.

SMOKING AND ORAL CARE

Tobacco smoking affects the prevalence and progression of many periodontal diseases. Smokers have greater pocket depths and bone and attachment loss compared with non-smokers. Tobacco products have direct effects on the periodontium and can alter the host response. Smokers respond less well to periodontal therapy.
Smoking is a risk factor for oral malignancy (e.g. squamous cell carcinoma).

The health of your patient may also have an influence on the type of care that is provided. Multiple, long appointments may not be suitable for patients in poor health. Many drugs cause dry mouth and this may either preclude certain types of treatment or affect the prognosis of treatment. Limited manual dexterity may mean that a patient may have problems maintaining particular types of restorations. It is important to realise that age will also have an impact as it can affect behaviour and the probability of disease. Older patients are more likely to have heavily restored dentitions and dentures. The elderly may have reduced mobility or may be unable to attend the surgery for care.

Clinical findings are not to be confused with a diagnosis. Dental caries is a clinical finding; dental caries owing to frequent sugar intakes (e.g. in tea) is a diagnosis. Remember that diagnosis is not merely detection and therefore the risk factors for the individual patient should be established as they must impact on the decision-making process.

Dentist factors

There are many influences on how we as dentists make decisions. We are influenced by what and by how we have been taught. Knowledge we have gained from clinical experience shapes our decision-making. If you have worked in a geographic area with a population that has high caries levels then that will affect the treatment you provide. Our own attitudes towards risk will influence the type of care that we are happy and willing to provide to individual patients. We also have our own values about dental health and a knowledge of our levels of skill. Clinical skills include decision-making abilities and communication skills as well as technical expertise. All of these take time to acquire and we must be pragmatic about our own abilities. Confidence in the skills that we have is also important and will influence patients' perceptions of our performance.

If you are unhappy about providing a treatment because of a lack of knowledge or skill or because you do not think it is the right treatment for the patient then you should not attempt to carry it out. Things will inevitably go wrong if you attempt treatment that you are not confident to provide, for whatever reason.

Risk assessment

Risk is inevitable in life and is impossible to avoid. Every individual has a different attitude to risk for specific events. One patient may be quite happy to have a general anaesthetic for a simple extraction despite having the risks explained, whereas another may refuse even local analgesia for the same procedure. Some patients will be more prepared to try a novel restorative material for which there is little scientific evidence than to have an amalgam restoration because they are so concerned about perceived risks associated with a dental material containing mercury.

It is important to assess each patient's attitude towards risk. You should also be aware of your own attitude and how this influences what you say to patients about possible treatment options. If your own third molar removal was extremely painful as the result of infection, you may discourage patients from having the same procedure. You may also be unsure of your own success at specific procedures and may over- or underestimate how well you perform in comparison with the average dentist.

Ideally of course we should not bring our personal perceptions into other people's care, but we have to accept that this is possible and is human nature. In order to assess risk for each patient it is important to work through a standard routine. This should involve an assessment of the risks involved and the probabilities of success for all the possible treatment options. This should be done from knowledge of the literature, such as systematic reviews or audits, and not just from past personal experiences. You should then be able to inform your patient about the risks involved in different treatment options and involve the patient in the decision-making process. To do the latter you must have assessed the patient's understanding and evaluation of your explanation and have come to a conclusion about their attitude towards risk and the value they place on the potential result of dental treatment.

There are very few medical or dental interventions that do not carry some risk, however in primary dental care these are normally very small. If this is the case, do we need to inform our patients of all the risks associated with every item of treatment we carry out? The obvious answer to that question is no, so what should we tell our patients? It is important to remember that consent to treatment is more than a simple agreement to treatment. It is also not merely warning a patient about the risks associated with care. For patients to give their consent to treatment they must have been given enough information about the proposed treatment, any possible alternatives and any substantial or special risks. All of this must be provided in a way that they can understand. Patients must also have the ability to understand the nature of treatment and the consequences of accepting, or declining, care. This ability is known as 'competence'. Finally they must not be coerced into care. Failure to give advice by explaining the options and the risks could be considered to be negligence.

Communication

If patients are to understand and appreciate the information about care, then we must be able to communicate this to them. We must take reasonable care to ensure that the explanations that we give are in a language that the individual patient can understand, and we must assess their level of understanding. Communication involves not only the actual spoken word but also the use of the tone of the voice to convey attitude and emotion and, most importantly, non-verbal communication or 'body language'. Other methods of communication include the use of illustrations, photographs, intra-oral cameras, study models and examples of laboratory work and information leaflets.

Poor communicators make poor clinicians as they cannot give the information in appropriate terms to their patients. Tailor your explanation to your audience. Listen to your patient: this is what they want you to do and it will allow you to learn about your patient and their understanding of their dental health. Many patients, particularly those who are unwell or vulnerable psychosocially, want a patient-centred approach, with communication, partnership and health promotion.

Cost of treatment

The cost of treatment is expressed not only in monetary terms but also in terms of social and emotional costs. Patients who are very anxious about dental treatment will not wish to 'spend' their emotional energy on a course of complex treatment. To such patients, the cost would be too high. This will also be the case for patients who have time restrictions on their attendance. To them, taking time off work for dental treatment may result in loss of earnings or in increased childcare costs, and the benefits are insufficient for such a personal sacrifice.

There are financial costs associated with each clinical option. These should form part of the information that you give to the patient when discussing the various options. It is not only the initial costs that need to be made clear, but also maintenance and replacement costs. One of the other factors related to cost is the longevity of any treatment option. This may simply mean advising a patient that you have provided with an immediate denture that this will require relining or replacement within a relatively short time (normally one year). A more complex explanation may be required when considering the choice between an amalgam and a gold restoration. A gold restoration may have higher initial costs but in statistical terms, it has a greater longevity.

Clinical factors

We will look at clinical choices in more detail in the next chapter, but here is an illustration of all the factors to be considered for one simple decision. The simplest decision may be thought to be that of whether to extract a tooth or to retain it. There are, however, many clinical factors that need to be taken into account when this decision is made. The options are usually to extract or to root treat the tooth, but the possibility of leaving the tooth without active treatment should also be considered. Many patients are happy with this last option, in the absence of pain or other symptoms.

Clinical factors to consider in the restore/extract decision:
- Can the tooth be restored? There is no point in carrying out root treatment on a tooth if the tooth cannot be restored in a satisfactory way. Even if you are considering the use of the tooth as an overdenture abutment, you must still be able to place a restoration. Extensive caries extending subgingivally or into the pulp chamber may mean that the tooth is not restorable, similarly for teeth with minimal amounts of tooth tissue remaining.

- Is root canal treatment possible? It is important to make careful assessment of the tooth before commencing root canal treatment as many factors may preclude successful treatment. These include: complicated root or canal anatomy, sclerosed canals or canals blocked with solid pastes, silver points, posts or separated instruments, persistent periradicular infection and inability to achieve a coronal seal. The technical quality of the final root treatment is not the only factor to influence the outcome of root canal treatment. Factors that may also be involved include the use of good isolation techniques such as rubber dam and the use of appropriate irrigants, for example sodium hypochlorite.
- Is there adequate bone support? The amount of bone support required will depend on the chosen restoration but the following may influence your decision: significant mobility (grade III), furcation involvement (grades II or III), loss of attachment of greater than 6 mm, bone loss of greater than 50% root length.
- Is the tooth important in the overall treatment plan? This perhaps is the most important question. This decision may be influenced by considerations of appearance; whether the tooth is important for the retention and support of a removable prosthesis, now or in the future; whether it is important to maintain the occlusion; or whether keeping this tooth would mean that a removable prosthesis would not be necessary. If you have worked out a strategy for treatment then this will be an easier question to answer.

DEVELOPING A TREATMENT STRATEGY

A strategy is a plan for achieving one's aims. A strategy for treatment allows you to manage care according to a long term plan. This means that every item of treatment is performed with an ultimate treatment objective in mind. To achieve this, priorities must be identified and then resources (time, money, skill) can be directed to those priorities. With long term goals you are not just dealing with problems as they arise. With a day-to-day management approach, goals are short term and usually related to the avoidance of extractions. The latter can work for younger patients with minimally restored dentitions and reasonable dental health, but is not suitable for patients with heavily restored dentitions, which almost inevitably will develop acute problems and decisions may need to be made quickly about specific treatment options. Recent surveys report that older adults have increased numbers of restorations, with 50% of the teeth of adults older than 45 years being filled or crowned. Trying to deal with problems in these patients on a short term basis does not encourage rational treatment decisions. A treatment strategy allows you to identify key teeth. Having done this you can concentrate resources in the correct direction. This may prevent your patient from requiring a removable prosthesis or it may stop you from having to preclude the possibility of further bridge work.

In order to develop a strategy you and your patient need to have decided the aims of treatment. In deciding on the objectives of treatment, a balance has to be achieved between the effort needed for treatment and the results obtained. It is important for your patient to realise that treatment may be changed or modified as a result of success or failure during the initial phase of care. They have an important impact on the success or otherwise of the care you wish to provide, as only they can modify their diet or oral hygiene habits.

Priorities in treatment

This may be a balance between patient and dentist as we may both have different priorities. This should be established before treatment is started. Normally the relief of pain is the first priority for the patient *and* the dentist (fig. 5.2). Pain is often the reason for initial attendance at the dental surgery. Fortunately, the relief of dental pain is normally possible assuming the correct diagnosis has been made. There may be rare cases when this is not achieved but normally this is due to misdiagnosis or the pain not being of dental origin. After the relief of pain, consideration should be given to the control of active disease. This will allow further assessment of the patient,

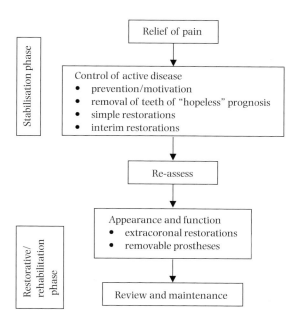

Figure 5.2 Order of treatment provision.

including their attitude towards care and their management and maintenance of their oral health. If active disease is not a priority for the patient,
then the options are to explain your reasons for managing disease or to
accept the patient's point of view. If your patient is getting married next week
and has fractured a central incisor, the caries in their molar teeth is not a priority to them – not unreasonably. Control of disease may involve a number of
treatment items. It should certainly include an appropriate preventive
regime. This may be dietary advice, oral hygiene instruction or smoking cessation therapy. At this stage any teeth that are of hopeless prognosis should
be extracted. Initial periodontal therapy including removal of plaque traps
such as ledges on restorations should be completed. This phase, which may
be termed the stabilisation phase, may also include root canal treatment,
simple direct restorations and the provision of interim dentures or indirect
restorations.

On completion of this stage, it is essential to review what has been
achieved and reassess the treatment plan. Assuming an appropriate level of
oral health has been achieved and maintained over a suitable time period, we
can then consider the appearance and functional needs and wishes of our
patients.

Treatment planning

The best treatment plan for any patient is normally the simplest interven-
tion(s) that adequately meet the needs, wants and abilities of the patient.

Treatment decision-making is not merely a case of deciding whether or
not to treat disease. There are many factors to be considered for each case and
many influences on how treatment is decided on for an individual patient. In
the next chapter we will look in more detail at clinical choices, but we should
not forget the other influences on care that have been discussed in this
chapter – to do so would result in poor treatment planning.

6 Clinical choices

INTRODUCTION

We discussed the influences on decision-making in the last chapter. One of those influences is the evidence base for different care options. In dentistry, there is limited 'scientific' evidence and many of our decisions may be based on clinical experience, either our own or that of other people. This may also be called clinical judgement. For each option, the evidence about that treatment should be considered, especially the advantages, disadvantages and the risks. There are very few medical or dental interventions that have no disadvantages or side effects.

It should always be remembered that doing nothing is an important option that may have fewer disadvantages or risks than other treatments. Patients may be content with the knowledge that their disease process is under control and not progressing. Or they may wish to have regular reviews before they commit to extensive dental care. The latter choice may also be yours as you may be unsure about the patient's response to the initial phase of management.

There are many possible care options for the same clinical condition. Patients present with a variety of clinical conditions, some of which may be more dominant in their mouths than others. Whatever the diagnosis there are usually several options for treatment and we need to know what these are and where and when to use them. The advantages, disadvantages and risks associated with each option must be known so that you and the patient can make informed choices about care. Treatment not only involves active restorative care but also prevention of disease.

SUPPORTING TISSUE MANAGEMENT

Periodontal diseases

The commonest inflammatory periodontal diseases are plaque-induced gingivitis and chronic periodontitis. Plaque-induced gingivitis is related to the patient's ability to maintain their oral hygiene. Motivating patients to improve their oral hygiene can be very difficult and you will not always succeed. We all know that we should not smoke, should exercise regularly and eat healthily but we often fail to do so. Patients frequently do not follow or comply with advice relating to their health. It has been estimated that between one-third and one half of all patients do not follow the medical advice given to them. Motivation is not the repetition of advice: you have to create a desire within your patient to change and you also have to understand what is concerning your patient and what they believe about their disease. Any advice should be relevant and realistic as well as specific, simple and short. Oral hygiene methods include tooth brushing methods, interproximal cleaning and the use of disclosing solutions or tablets. Removal of calculus and ledges on restorations will help your patient with their oral hygiene, as can a professional prophylaxis. It makes the mouth feel clean and is usually a pleasant dental procedure for patients. Repeating plaque and bleeding scores allows you to keep an objective measure of your patient's progress with oral hygiene and can be used to motivate. Your patient has an essential role in controlling their gingival condition. If this is not controlled it can affect your treatment planning as it would be imprudent to carry out complex restorative treatment in a patient who, for whatever reason, is unable to maintain good oral hygiene.

Between 10 and 20 per cent of the population is susceptible to destructive periodontal disease. Most periodontal disease is initiated by dental plaque but may be complicated by systemic factors, such as diabetes, or by local factors such as poorly contoured restorations.

The management of chronic periodontitis involves the identification of local and systemic factors, the extraction of teeth with hopeless prognosis, improving oral hygiene, root debridement, possible use of antimicrobial adjuncts, monitoring and reassessment at 6–12 weeks. Surgery may be necessary to gain access to root surfaces for thorough debridement.

Common mucosal problems

Chronic atrophic candidiasis (denture stomatitis)

This affects between a quarter and two-thirds of denture-wearers and is more common in females. It has several causative factors:
• Trauma from dentures
• Presence of *Candida Albicans* or other *Candida* species
• Systemic factors.
Before any new denture is made this condition should be treated because the tissues will be swollen. If impressions are taken without resolving the candidiasis, the swelling will be duplicated in the new denture. Inflammation then resolves under the new denture, resulting in lack of fit, and a causative factor is re-established. Treatment involves reducing the denture trauma, leaving the denture out at night and improving denture hygiene. The use of topical antifungal agents such as amphotericin, nystatin or miconazole should be considered if local measures do not bring about resolution. If none of these measures resolves the candidiasis, consider the possibility of an underlying systemic problem and refer the patient to his/her general medical practitioner.

Flabby ridge

This is classically seen under a complete upper denture opposed by natural lower anterior teeth. The unbalanced occlusion results in resorption of the alveolar bone, which is then replaced by fibrous tissue. Stability of the denture is compromised as a result of the fibrous tissue. For flabby ridges you need to use an impression technique that will not displace the tissues. If the fibrous tissue is distorted, the new denture will fit only when seated by occlusal pressure. When the teeth are apart, elastic recoil of the displaced tissue forces the denture downwards. The new denture should be made on a model cast from an impression of the flabby ridge in its resting position. Your impression technique should involve a material of low viscosity and a spaced tray, possibly perforated as well.

Traumatic ulcers

Traumatic ulcers may develop within one and two days of denture insertion or in association with a fractured tooth or rough area of a restoration. Healing should occur within a few days of the correction of the problem and if this does not occur then another diagnosis must be considered.

REPAIR OF TEETH

Teeth may require repair as the result of dental caries, tooth wear, trauma or developmental defects. Despite decreases in the occurrence of primary dental caries in most industrialised countries, the restoration of teeth continues to be necessary. Maintenance and replacement of existing restorations represent a large component of this dental treatment, particularly in the older adult.

A number of factors have to be taken into account when choosing the most appropriate restorative method and material for a clinical situation. The limiting factors include:
• Patient motivation and suitability
• The number of remaining teeth and their relative positions
• The condition of the supporting tissues
• The amount of remaining tooth structure
• The restorative materials available, and their longevity as restoratives
• The occlusion and opposing teeth and restorations
• Aesthetic and other wishes of the patient, including cost factors.
When any method or material is chosen, it must be used in the most appropriate clinical situation.

Dental caries

Prevention

Dental caries is a preventable disease. The carious process may be modified in a number of ways:
• Diet modification – reducing the frequency of sugar intake and limiting it to mealtimes is a very effective way to prevent dental caries.
• Fluoride – the use of appropriate levels of fluoride will delay caries progress. Fluoride sources include water supply, toothpaste, mouthwashes and professionally applied sources such as gel or varnish.
• Plaque control – removal of plaque traps and advice to patients about maintaining good oral hygiene are vital components of caries management.
• Xerostomia – patients with dry mouth through low saliva levels are more prone to dental caries and will require advice about how this can be managed.
• Fissure sealants – these resins can render a tooth less susceptible to fissure and pit caries.

Restorative management

There is currently a debate about whether dental caries should be removed fully or partially from a cavity or whether it should be sealed in place. Evidence suggests that sealing over caries will arrest the process. Fissure sealants placed over occlusal caries extending into the middle third of dentine will arrest the lesion. For grossly carious cavities, stepwise excavation may be used. Caries is removed in two steps, 6–12 months apart. At the first visit access is gained, caries is removed from the periphery only, leaving soft caries on the cavity floor. The cavity is restored with calcium hydroxide and sealed with glass ionomer. At the subsequent visit, on re-entry into the cavity the dentine is found to be harder and drier with fewer micro-organisms present. Another technique is ultraconservative caries removal. It involves preparing the tooth minimally by cutting a 1 mm bevel in the sound enamel surrounding the cavitated lesion. No further preparation is carried out and the tooth is restored with acid-etch retained composites and fissure sealant. This technique has been used successfully to arrest occlusal caries.

Dental caries may be removed in a number of ways other than the conventional use of burs in a handpiece or by hand instruments. Chemomechanical removal involves the use of a gel which softens the collagen in the carious tissue through chlorination of amino acids, thus allowing easy mechanical removal with specially designed hand instruments. Air abrasion employs alumina particles in a high velocity stream of air to remove tooth substance. For both these techniques local analgesia may not be required but they are time-consuming and with air abrasion there is limited tactile sensation. Lasers for hard tissue removal have yet to achieve full acceptance.

Available materials

There are many materials available for the intracoronal restoration of carious cavities. The direct restoratives in current, general use are amalgam, composite, glass ionomer and combinations of the last two groups. Indirect restorations in cast metal, composite and ceramic are also possible.

Dental amalgam continues to be used despite concerns about health and the environment because it has high clinical success, known performance, relatively low cost and is easy to manipulate. Despite the high usage of this material it is not ideal and suffers from several problems including marginal breakdown, fracture and poor appearance. Secondary caries is the most common reason given for the replacement of amalgam restorations but this diagnosis may not necessarily always be correct. There is a well-recognised need for effective alternatives, not least because of its less than ideal properties but also because of public and political concerns about its use, the changing patterns of dental disease and patient expectations of dental care.

Direct resin composites are the material of choice for anterior intracoronal restorations and they are increasing in use and popularity for posterior intracoronal restorations, mainly because of their appearance. The physical characteristics of these materials are much improved from their initial forms, and methods of handling them have developed considerably and are no longer copies of amalgam techniques. However, it can be more difficult to generate good proximal contour and contact with these materials. Polymerisation shrinkage of the resin during curing still occurs and may contribute to marginal defects, cuspal distortion or crack formation in the enamel or dentine and may therefore contribute to post-operative sensitivity for the patient. There are a number of clinical techniques available to overcome these problems and the longevity of restorations of the newer resin composites is much improved over that of the original materials. The principal use of these materials in posterior teeth should be limited to small to medium-sized restorations, for example in premolar teeth with little occlusal function or in areas of molars that are not supporting the occlusion. They may also be used successfully for core build-ups to support laboratory fabricated crown and bridge work.

Glass ionomers contain poly(alkenoic) acid and fluoroaluminosilicate glass which set by an acid-base reaction to give a cement. They adhere directly to tooth substance and to base metal casting alloys. They release fluoride after placement giving the materials cariostatic properties, although this may only be short term. They also have a low tensile strength which makes them brittle and unsuitable for use in load-bearing areas in permanent teeth. They are used as lining and luting materials and to restore abrasion and erosion lesions, Class V cavities, and deciduous teeth and as interim restorations. It must be appreciated however that they are less translucent than resin composite restoratives and therefore their appearance is less good.

Resin modified glass ionomers have a resin (monomer) component as well as the poly(alkenoic) acid and fluoroaluminosilicate glass of conventional glass ionomers. They set by two mechanisms, namely an acid-base reaction and curing of the monomer (chemically, by light or both). They have improved appearance and physical properties compared with conventional glass ionomers. They are used in similar situations to glass ionomers and may also be used for small core build-ups.

Compomers are polyacid-modified resin composites. Their properties are more like those of composites than glass ionomers. They have limited fluoride release but are stronger and have a better appearance than glass ionomers. Their wear resistance is less than that of composite restoratives. They do not adhere directly to tooth substance without the use of a bonding system. They may be utilised to restore Class V and Class III cavities and for deciduous teeth.

Cast metal inlays have a very substantial reputation for longevity in clinical service, stability of anatomic form and long-term retention of marginal characteristics and surface finish. In situations where an onlay or inlay is indicated, where there are no requirements to use a tooth-coloured restorative and stability of anatomic form is of importance, a cast metal inlay or onlay of high precious metal content has many advantages. The longevity of gold restorations exceeds that of any current alternatives by a factor of two to four. Cast metal is strong in thin section and depending on which alloy is used, is slightly ductile allowing the margins of the restoration to be burnished to improve fit. Cast metal is a very versatile material. The indirect technique allows it to be shaped to restore contours and contact areas. Setting aside the appearance of cast metal restorations (as not all patients consider this a disadvantage), the other principal limitations of such restorations may be overcome with the further development and acceptance of surface treatments and resin bonded luting systems for cast metal restorations.

Ceramics have favourable biocompatibility and good appearance. They have good wear resistance characteristics and are inert in the oral environment. The development of stronger ceramics and improved luting techniques have resulted in ceramic inlays and onlays becoming realistic alternatives to cast metal restorations. Reported problems with these restorations include fragile occlusal margins, marginal fit, and bulk fracture. They can also be difficult to adjust and must be polished following any adjustments to prevent wear of the opposing teeth. The inertness of the material means that surface treatments such as etching and silane application are necessary to achieve a good bond to tooth substance. High alumina products have therefore to be sand-blasted rather than etched.

Material retention

Several techniques may be used to aid the retention of the restorative material. Retention and resistance form is important for non-adhesive direct and indirect restorations. Removal of primary caries creates an undercut cavity that aids retention of direct materials. Additional retention for non-adhesive materials may be gained by cutting slots, grooves or boxes. Pins have been used extensively in the past but they have many disadvantages: they are difficult to place and seat and their incorrect placement can result in perforation through the root side into the periodontal ligament space or in pulpal exposure. They can also cause tooth fracture. Their use has decreased substantially with the increased use of other methods of retaining restoratives.

Acid etching creates pores within enamel into which resin flows to create tags. This micromechanical retention is very reliable unless there has been contamination of the etched surface by saliva or blood. Bonding to dentine may be achieved reliably with current systems involving one or two steps and which remove or modify the smear layer. Amalgam can be bonded to the cavity using adhesive resins. The potential advantages of this technique are reduced sensitivity and marginal leakage, the reduced need for mechanical cavity retentive features and improved strength of the restored tooth. At present there is a paucity of information on the long-term clinical outcome of this technique.

Heavily restored teeth

Large direct restorations can be difficult to carry out well as access to deep boxes may be awkward and handling a large bulk of material is not easy. It can be difficult to recreate the dental anatomy, especially the contact areas, occlusal contour and the marginal ridges. Failure rates for large restorations are higher than for small restorations and once one cusp of a posterior tooth has been replaced, an indirect restoration with cuspal coverage should be considered.

Another reason to consider replacing a large direct restoration with an indirect one is when the tooth is root-treated. Root treatment does not make a tooth inherently brittle, however the removal of tooth substance, particularly the roof of the pulp chamber and the marginal ridges, weakens the tooth. For posterior teeth, if both marginal ridges have been broken, a restoration covering the occlusal surface is indicated. This could be a cuspal coverage amalgam or a cast metal restoration. Removal of large amounts of dentine from the axial wall for a crown preparation (particularly metal ceramic crowns) further weakens a tooth and therefore consideration should be given to partial coverage crowns or cuspal coverage onlays. Root treated posterior teeth that have not been restored with a crown are more prone to dental caries and therefore it is important to provide restorations with good marginal fit and smooth surfaces to minimise plaque accumulation.

Extracoronal restorations

There are several types of crowns. They may be described by the materials from which they are constructed and by the amount of coronal coverage.

Gold is the best of the currently available materials for crowns. The only disadvantage is its appearance and this may not be a consideration for all patients. It is normally used for posterior teeth only, is easy to adjust and can be used in thin section allowing for minimal amounts of tooth substance removal. Gold crowns are adaptable as it is easy to change the shape of a tooth or incorporate features such as rest seats or undercuts for clasps to help in the support and retention of a partial denture. Gold has a hardness similar to that of enamel and wears at a similar rate to enamel.

There are several types of all ceramic crowns. The porcelain jacket crown (PJC) is the commonest type although this may be superseded by the resin bonded crown. PJCs are only really suitable for anterior teeth as the material is brittle. They require an even amount of tooth substance removal (approximately 1 mm axially) to ensure support for the crown. High strength ceramics have been used for posterior teeth but these require substantially greater tooth preparation.

Resin bonded crowns are full coverage ceramic restorations that are bonded to the tooth using a resin composite luting system. Such crowns have good fracture resistance once bonded and require minimal preparation. They can be used where there has already been tooth substance loss or where there is limited remaining crown height. They are often used in cases of tooth substance loss by erosion. Their appearance can be excellent although this may be compromised if care is not taken over the luting stage. This procedure is technique sensitive and time consuming compared with conventional crowns and it should be noted that at present there are no long term clinical results on these restorations.

Metal ceramic (porcelain fused to metal) crowns may be used anteriorly and posteriorly. They have good strength and can have excellent appearance. They require more tooth substance removal than cast metal crowns and if tooth reduction is inadequate from the axial walls, appearance and shape can be compromised resulting in opaque, over-contoured restorations. Tooth reduction occlusally can be minimised by designing the crown to have a metal occlusal surface. This improves retention and resistance and is easier to fabricate in the laboratory and to adjust at the chairside and negates the possibility of a rough occlusal ceramic surface damaging the opposing teeth.

A post is used to retain a core which supports a crown. Posts do not strengthen teeth and should be avoided where there is adequate remaining tooth tissue to retain a crown without the need for a post. Parallel sided posts are retained better than tapering posts; however in very tapering root canals, a parallel sided post may result in excess dentine removal. Posts may be fabricated in the laboratory or may be supplied ready made. Laboratory-made posts are made from cast metal and may involve the use of pre-formed elements, such as plastic burn-out posts. Ready-made posts are metal or fibre and require the addition of a core in a plastic material. Cores may be made from amalgam, composite or resin-modified glass ionomer. The latter is more suitable for small amounts of tooth build-up.

Risks

All restorations have sequelae for the teeth involved. A number of factors are thought to influence the likelihood of a tooth becoming non-vital following dental treatment. These include the preoperative condition of the tooth, the cutting temperature and duration of any tooth preparation, the use of local analgesia and retraction cord, the length of time of temporisation and the area of exposed root surface. To reduce the risk of loss of vitality following tooth preparation, the following may help:

• Remove infected dentine
• Proper cooling and preparation design
• A well-fitting temporary crown
• Cement the permanent crown as soon as possible.

Loss of pulp vitality can occur following crown preparation. Histological studies demonstrate pulp reactions to dental treatment. The incidence and risk period of pulp deterioration following crown preparation remain uncertain as a number of cross-sectional studies have shown differing results. From theses studies, the approximate mean value for periapical changes on teeth restored with crowns or bridges is 10 per cent at 10 years. Longevity for crowns is also influenced by other factors such as caries rates, gingival recession, and porcelain fracture.

Failure rates are high for post retained crowns. Loss of retention may occur owing to inadequate post length or design or to vertical root fracture. Perforation is also a risk of post crowns.

Toothwear

Preventive advice

This obviously depends on the diagnosis of the type of tooth surface loss (which can be difficult – see Chapter 4) and the specific cause. If erosive tooth surface loss caused by food or drink is the diagnosis then advice regarding substitution with something less erosive should be given. Carbonated drinks are a common cause of dental erosion and the appropriate advice would be to substitute these drinks with less acidic drinks, such as water, tea, coffee, milk and to restrict intake of acidic drinks to meal times. If you suspect that an eating disorder may be the cause of the erosive tooth surface loss, it is important to try and ensure that the patient seeks help, as early diagnosis and treatment can dramatically alter the course of the disease and the patient's long-term welfare. Discussions about such issues with patients should aim to reach an agreement about how best to proceed. Other medical conditions such as hiatus hernia may also require medical referral if this is not already in place. There are many other causes of erosive tooth surface loss such as excess vitamin C intake or specific occupations: examples of these include wine tasters and historically, battery factory workers. It is difficult to suggest that someone gives up his or her livelihood and advice must therefore be tailored to the individual patient.

The commonest cause of abrasion is poor tooth brushing technique. Advice should concentrate on choice of brush and paste and brushing technique. Attrition that is pathological, as opposed to physiological, may be the result of a highly abrasive diet or parafunction. Making the patient aware of the cause is an important first step. If parafunction is the cause then careful assessment of the occlusion is important. It may be appropriate to supply a soft splint to prevent further damage to the teeth. In specific cases, attrition may be the result of wear from poorly finished ceramic restorations and these should either be polished or replaced.

Monitoring

This can be an important stage in managing tooth wear as a definitive diagnosis may not have been possible and even if it has been, it is useful to assess whether the advice given has had any affect. Monitoring should involve looking for signs and symptoms of continuing wear. These are not only the physical tooth surface loss but also signs such as tongue scalloping and cheek ridging that indicate a grinding habit or the accumulation of stain that may suggest that an erosive habit has ceased. Physical tooth wear may be monitored clinically by the use of study models, photographs and silicone indices. Mouthguards may be used in the management of toothwear. If patients grind their teeth they can grind the mouthguard instead. This may also interrupt the habit as well as being diagnostic of the cause of toothwear and protective of the tooth substance. The mouthguard may be made from soft or hard acrylic for the mandibular or maxillary teeth but should always be full coverage as partial coverage will allow over-eruption of the uncovered teeth.

Restorative treatment

Restorative treatment of tooth substance loss may be required for a number of reasons. These include sensitivity, poor appearance and concern regarding the long term prognosis. Protection of the teeth may be required to prevent further tissue loss.

Sensitivity from exposed dentine is thought to be due to movement of fluid in the dentinal tubules. Obturating the tubules should prevent the symptoms of sensitivity. Management of dental sensitivity in tooth substance loss cases should involve removal, reduction or modification of the aetiological factors. Some improvement may be obtained from the use of a desensitising toothpaste. Prescription of a fluoride mouth rinse, once daily for a month may offer additional relief. If teeth do not respond to this approach then a resin composite or resin-modified glass ionomer may be applied to the affected teeth.

The usual concern relating to poor appearance of the teeth is that they are becoming shorter. Short teeth can be difficult to restore as they are inherently unretentive. There are, however a number of techniques available to manage such situations. Crown lengthening surgery, orthodontics to extrude the tooth, or elective root canal treatment may be carried out. Appropriate restorations may be chosen and designed to account for the lack of mechanical retention in the remaining tooth structure. Adhesive restorations such as direct resin composites may be utilised or indirect restorations such as composites and ceramics or sand-blasted gold, luted with an appropriate composite luting agent, may be fabricated. Alternatively the short teeth may be made into overdenture abutments or restored with an overlay denture.

Lack of space between opposing teeth to allow for restorations may be a problem. Further removal of tooth substance to provide space for restorations may result in pulpal exposure or may reduce the teeth to a height that could not reasonably retain a restoration. Lack of space occurs because of compensatory alveolar growth and the teeth are still in contact despite the loss of inter-occlusal tooth substance.

Space for restorations is therefore required. In general terms, such space may be gained by:
• Increasing the occluso-vertical dimension (OVD).
• Orthodontic treatment.
• Using the difference between centric occlusion and centric relation.

Increasing OVD may be achieved in a number of ways:

- Resin composite may be applied to cover worn surfaces and build up incisal edges or occlusal surfaces. Such restorations have the advantages of being relatively simple and quick and of requiring minimal tooth preparation. They are reversible yet provide an immediate improvement in appearance. They are also easy to repair and are relatively inexpensive (figs 6.1a and b).
- Extracoronal restorations such as cast metal, ceramic or indirect composite onlays or crowns may be used. These will normally require some form of additional devices to achieve retention to the short clinical crowns. This may take the form of grooves or boxes in the preparation or the use of dentine bonding systems and surface preparation of the restorations.
- Dentures, in the form of partial overlay or overdentures, are another method of increasing the OVD. Additions to existing dentures can help the patient adjust to this change.

For anterior tooth wear, the commonest type of orthodontic treatment is the use of an anterior bite plane. This separates the posterior teeth and allows alveolar compensation in the posterior segments and results in space behind

(a)
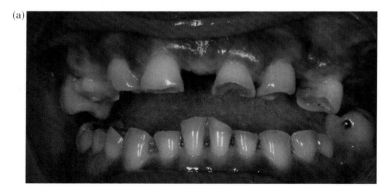

(b)
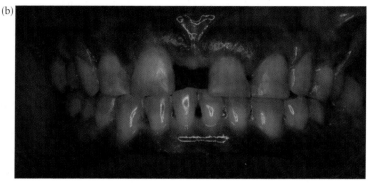

Figure 6.1 (a) and (b) Composite for toothwear.

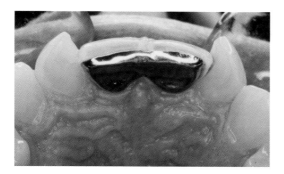

Figure 6.2 Dahl appliance.

the upper anterior teeth that may be used for placing a restoration to cover the palatal surfaces. In restorative dentistry this is known as the 'Dahl principle'. Dahl appliances were originally removable and made of cobalt chrome. These have been superseded by fixed alternatives which may be made of cobalt chrome, silver, composite resin or ceramic (fig 6.2). Dahl appliances normally work within six to nine months. The palatal tooth surfaces may subsequently be restored directly with composite or indirectly with gold or ceramic veneers or with resin-bonded crowns.

Another method of obtaining space for restorations is utilising the difference between centric occlusion and centric relation. When teeth or tooth substance is lost posteriorly, patients may posture their mandible forward to a more anterior centric occlusion. If their mandible is allowed to go back towards centric relation, then there may be space available for the restoration of the worn teeth.

Trauma

Management of trauma is important. Trauma usually involves the upper incisors and the loss of these teeth can be very upsetting for patients and can result in the need for extensive dental treatment.

Pulpal complications are rare following simple crown fracture without pulpal involvement, but will increase if a luxation injury is involved. If pulpal exposure has occurred then treatment with pulp capping or partial pulpotomy will increase the chance of pulp survival. A direct pulp cap is more likely to be successful if pulp exposure is small and treatment is provided within 24 hours of the accident but pulp necrosis is common following luxation injuries to teeth with closed apices.

Avulsion should be managed immediately by reimplantation and use of a functional (not rigid) splint, such as resin composite, for 7–10 days. The aim of the splint is to stabilise the tooth in the bony socket to allow the periodontal ligament to reattach to bone and cementum root surface and for gingival fibres to reattach at the cervical margin of the tooth. The splint should allow some normal tooth movement within the socket to avoid ankylosis. The pulp remains vital in 30 per cent of avulsion cases after five years. Vitality depends on the size of the apex, the time the root surface is exposed, and how the tooth was stored. In teeth with closed apices, the pulp should be extirpated and a non-setting calcium hydroxide dressing placed to change local pH and induce osteoblasts to lay down new osteoid material. The canal should be filled with gutta percha 6–12 months later.

The management of root fracture depends on the location of the fracture. If it is close to the gingival margin then the coronal portion should be removed and an assessment made as to whether it is possible to root treat and restore the tooth using a post-retained restoration. It may be possible to extrude the root orthodontically to aid the placement of a crown. Fractures that are in the middle or apical third of the root should be splinted rigidly for three months. Root fractures heal by connective tissue, whereas non-healing involves granulation tissue. Pulpal necrosis occurs in approximately one quarter of cases, in which case the pulp should be extirpated to the fracture line and managed as for avulsion cases.

DENTINE HYPERSENSITIVITY

In most cases of dentine hypersensitivity, some improvement will be obtained from the use of a desensitising toothpaste containing potassium nitrate. The prescription of a sodium fluoride mouthrinse, once daily for a month, may offer additional relief. If the teeth do not respond to this approach then a resin composite or resin-modified glass ionomer may be applied to the exposed areas of dentine.

PULP MANAGEMENT

Pulpal inflammation can be the result of a number of causes and these include dental caries, tooth wear, trauma and dental treatment. This may lead to reversible or irreversible pulpitis or may result in a non-vital tooth with a necrotic pulp. Treatment of reversible pulpitis involves identifying the initiating factor, removing it if possible and restoring the tooth as necessary. Irreversible pulpitis will not resolve with any of these treatment options. Root canal treatment or extraction are the only treatment options. The causative factor must also be identified for apical (periradicular) periodontitis and this can result from pulpal inflammation, problems associated with root canal treatment or may simply be due to a high restoration. Treatment may involve occlusal adjustment, root canal treatment, periapical surgery or extraction.

Assessment of the condition of the pulp involves careful examination of the tooth and its surrounding tissues, sensitivity tests, and radiographs (see Chapter 2). You are not only assessing the condition of the pulp but also making decisions about possible treatment options. If the pulp is irreversibly damaged, you need to know whether it is possible to carry out root canal treatment *and* whether it is possible to restore the tooth *and* maintain it within the dentition.

The options for a non-vital tooth are to root treat it, extract it or leave it *in situ*. The latter option is often not mentioned but should always be considered, particularly in situations where root treatment is not possible or in cases where the patient does not wish treatment, despite being advised of the possible sequelae. It could possibly be an option when active treatment is not advisable – perhaps for medical reasons.

Root treatment may be conventional orthograde or surgical retrograde. It should be remembered that it is not only the quality of the final obturation that affects prognosis of root canal treatment but also other factors such as moisture control, infection control, disinfection, size of original apical lesion and the final seal. The final obturation should ideally be within 1 mm of the radiographic apex and well condensed. Longitudinal *controlled* studies of root canal treatments have shown that the peak incidence of healing is at one year, as is the peak incidence of emerging chronic apical periodontitis. At one year, almost 90 per cent of the teeth that heal eventually, demonstrate signs of healing and reversal of the healing process is rare. Unfortunately, in cross-sectional studies the success rate is much lower, sometimes as low as 60 per cent.

If an apical area is seen on radiograph in relation to an existing RCT, should the root treatment be redone? This is a controversial area and a judgement must be made. Factors that will influence you to redo the root treatment include an increasing size of periapical area, a root treatment that has been unsealed for some time and the type of final restoration that is to be placed. If you are about to place a crown on this tooth, then consider whether there is a coronal seal or lining or a post, and whether the tooth is more difficult to re-root treat if it is restored with a crown.

REPLACEMENT OF TEETH

If a tooth is missing or extracted do we always need to replace it? The reasons that are usually quoted for replacing missing teeth are appearance and function. Appearance is a very personal thing and whereas one patient may be concerned about the appearance following the loss of an upper first molar tooth, another patient may not be. Personal preference, smile line, concerns about replacement options and concerns about having dental treatment carried out all contribute to a patient's decision-making processes.

Function is less often mentioned by patients than is appearance. The shortened dental arch is a type of treatment plan orientated towards function. Treatment goals are limited to preserving the anterior and premolar dentition. This technique provides a suboptimal but acceptable level of oral function. Careful case selection is required as there must be a good prognosis for the remaining teeth.

Simple

Options for replacing small numbers of missing teeth are:
- Accept the space
- Orthodontic treatment to close the space
- Resin retained bridge
- Conventional bridge
- Removable prosthesis
- Immediate denture
- Implant retained fixed restoration.

Specific factors to take into account when considering such replacement include the longevity of the different options, the possibility of retrieval if an option fails, the available designs, the patient's occlusion, the condition of the rest of the dentition and supporting tissues and the ability of the patient to maintain the restoration.

Complex

Options for replacing a larger number of teeth are:
- Removable prostheses
- Copy dentures
- Implant retained removable restorations
- Bridgework

Partial dentures/removable prostheses

These may be used as an interim restoration before the provision of a bridge or an implant or may be the definitive restoration. Partial dentures may also be utilised as a transition to over-dentures or complete dentures. There are many different types and designs of partial dentures, but most frameworks are fabricated from either cobalt chrome or acrylic. The choice will depend on the condition of the remaining dentition, the number, position and type of retained teeth, the occlusion and the overall plan for the dentition. Patient preference should also be considered. All-acrylic dentures are light, can have good appearance and can be added to following any further extractions. They need to have bulk for adequate strength and this may result in excessive mucosal coverage. Cobalt chrome dentures are strong in thin section and the design can incorporate clasps and rest seats and can cover less mucosa than

PARTIAL DENTURES

ADVANTAGES	DISADVANTAGES
• Can replace teeth, soft tissue and bone • Minimal tooth preparation, if any • Other options still possible as little or no tooth preparation • Replace multiple teeth, in different areas of arch • Support from mucosa and/or teeth • Appearance can be good • Least expensive • Can be designed to allow for future additions	• Increased dental plaque can result in caries and gingival problems • Coverage of the palate is often unpopular with patients – complaints regarding loss of taste relate to temperature and texture of food • The removable aspect not liked by patients, in general, owing to social concerns • Appearance compromised by clasps • Limited longevity which may negate lower initial cost

acrylic dentures. Mechanical interlocking is required for the addition of the acrylic components.

Resin retained bridges

The design most likely to succeed is a single cantilever (fig. 6.3). Double abutments and fixed–fixed designs should be avoided as they are more likely to fail. Before providing a resin retained bridge the following factors should be taken into account: spacing, occlusion, restoration of adjacent teeth, bone support, numbers of other teeth present, condition of mouth. There are a number of different fitting surface treatments for resin retained bridges but the common types are sand-blasting and acid or electrolytic etching. The Rochette bridge relies on mechanical retention from holes in the framework and still has a limited role as an interim restoration, perhaps during implant work. Resin retained components can be used in combination with conventional bridgework but you must allow for failure in the design by incorporating a movable joint so that when the resin retained component debonds, that part of the bridge may then be removed and rebonded. Success rate of resin retained bridges can be high but careful attention must be paid to design, surface treatment and adhesion.

Conventional bridgework

Conventional bridgework is often of a fixed–fixed design but may also be a cantilever, fixed–movable or a combination of elements. Common design examples are:

• Cantilever design – the replacement of an upper lateral incisor from the adjacent upper canine.

(a)

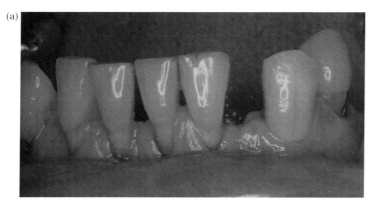

(b)

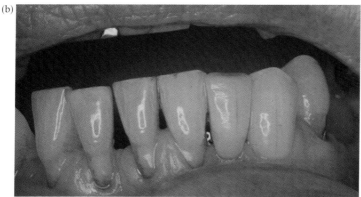

Figure 6.3 Resin retained bridge replacing LL2.

RESIN-RETAINED BRIDGEWORK

ADVANTAGES	DISADVANTAGES
• Minimal tooth preparation required depending on occlusion	• Not possible in many cases
• Fixed/not removable – patients like this aspect – also better for gingival health than partial denture	• Failure of retention – debond
	• Longevity limited
	• Technique sensitive
• Appearance can be good – may be compromised by metal wing show through	• Metal work of retainer may compromise appearance
• Failure – loss and caries – minimised if single cantilever	• What happens if any existing restoration fails under wing?

- Fixed–fixed – replacing a lower first permanent molar with the second permanent molar and second premolar as retainers.
- Fixed–movable – where abutment teeth are not parallel, for example a tilted lower molar.

CONVENTIONAL BRIDGEWORK

ADVANTAGES	DISADVANTAGES
• Fixed • Appearance can be good • Can incorporate changes to occlusion and appearance • Predictable	• Tooth preparation • Pulpal health compromised • Failure – mechanical and biological • Long spans have higher failure rates • High levels of skill – technical and clinical required • Irreversible

IMPLANT RETAINED PROSTHESES

ADVANTAGES	DISADVANTAGES
• Fixed or removable • Highly predictable • Longevity • Maintains bone	• Depend on amount and quality of bone • Surgery involved • Technique sensitive • Expensive – in money and time • High levels of maintenance required • Smoking can dramatically affect success and prognosis

OVERDENTURES

ADVANTAGES	DISADVANTAGES
• Bone retained • Proprioception • Psychological aspects • Transition to complete dentures	• Caries on root surfaces • Bulky • Difficult to maintain

The success rate is higher for short span bridges involving either the anterior region or the posterior regions of the mouth. Failure increases with length of span and for bridges involving both anterior and posterior teeth.

Implant retained prostheses

Implants are not primary dental care but they should be considered as a possible option to replace missing teeth and it is important to be able to outline their advantages and disadvantages to patients and to know where to access such secondary care.

Overdentures

Overdentures may be complete or partial and are made to cover roots which support the prosthesis. The advantages of overdentures over conventional dentures are the maintenance of alveolar bone, improved stability and retention from the retained bone, enhanced proprioception from the periodontal ligament and therefore improved masticatory ability for the patient, and the psychological aspects related to the retention of the roots of teeth. Disease control is important in overdenture cases as otherwise the root faces will rapidly decay. The ideal complete overdenture case has a minimum of two roots, symmetrically distributed in the mouth and with a dome-shaped crown. There should be at least 50 per cent bone support and root canal treatment should be possible.

MANAGING DISCOLOURED TEETH

Discolouration is usually classified as intrinsic or extrinsic. Smoking, red wine, coffee, tea, chlorhexidine or chromogenic bacteria may cause extrinsic staining. The common causes of intrinsic staining or mottling in vital teeth are tetracycline, fluoride, and inherited or acquired disorders. In non-vital teeth discolouration is the result of pulpal haemorrhage following trauma, pulpal necrosis or root canal treatment. The options for management depend on the diagnosis but include professional cleaning, home cleaning, bleaching, microabrasion and veneers.

Bleaching for vital teeth

This technique involves the use of agents that contain or produce hydrogen peroxide. It is commonly delivered in a gel form that is applied in mouth guards and worn at night for a few weeks, hence the term night guard bleaching. The gel is normally 10 per cent carbamide peroxide, although increased strengths may be used for a quick start to the bleaching process. Patients may report sensitivity using this technique and the outcome and prognosis is unpredictable. It is more likely to work in patients who have teeth that are towards the darker end of the shade guide. Tetracycline staining will take much longer to lighten. The use of such gels is currently illegal in the UK.

Bleaching non-vital teeth

Discolouration of non-vital teeth may be due to pulpal haemorrhage following trauma, incomplete removal of pulpal tissue when root canal treatment is carried out, or rarely, root canal cements or restorative materials may cause discolouration. Discolouration is seen in approximately 10 per cent of anterior teeth following root canal treatment. Bleaching techniques include walking bleach, thermocatalytic bleaching and inside/outside bleaching and is 90 per cent successful over five years. The technique can be repeated if

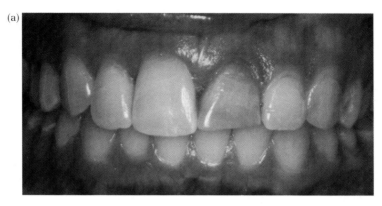

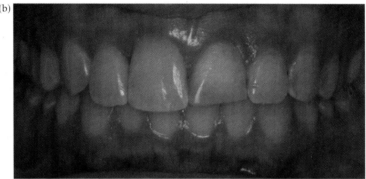

Figure 6.4 (a) and (b) Non-vital bleaching.

discolouration recurs. Possible complications include cervical resorption and crown fracture (figs 6.4a and b).

BLEACHING NON-VITAL TEETH

METHOD:

- Ensure that existing root canal treatment is adequate by checking radiographically
- Remove gutta percha to cement-enamel level
- Seal over gutta percha e.g. with a resin modified glass ionomer
- For walking bleach, place paste in pulp chamber e.g. sodium perborate (Bocasan) and water, then seal chamber with a small pledget of cotton wool and a temporary dressing
- Repeat at weekly intervals as necessary (usually two or three times)
- Rinse out all bleaching agent and restore tooth with resin composite

(a)

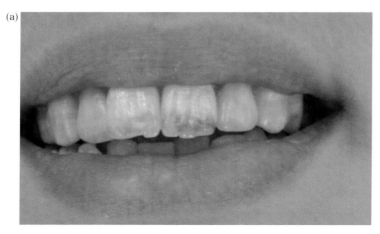

(b)

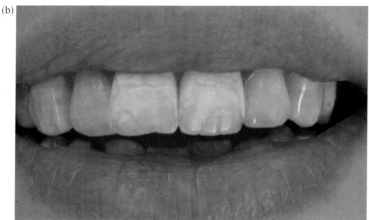

Figure 6.5 (a) and (b) Microabrasion.

Enamel microabrasion

This technique uses an acidified abrasive paste to produce removal of superficial enamel layers. It is used in the management of mottling caused by fluorosis. The technique is unpredictable but can be very successful (figs 6.5a and b).

Veneers

Teeth may be veneered directly using resin composite or indirectly by laboratory-made ceramic or resin composite veneers. Laboratory ceramic veneers can give extremely good results in respect of appearance and tooth shape but will involve some tooth preparation and careful examination of the occlusion

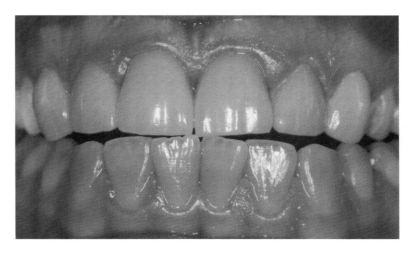

Figure 6.6 Porcelain veneers on the upper anterior teeth.

is essential. The appearance from composite veneers can be good initially but they will require finishing and polishing on a regular basis and as such may be an interim restoration. Temporisation for laboratory veneers can be difficult and definitive luting requires great care and attention to detail. Careful choice of luting cements will allow differing amounts of discolouration to be masked. Veneers are usually used in the management of discoloured upper anterior teeth as occlusal relationships and the size of the lower incisors may preclude their use in the mandible (fig. 6.6).

CONCLUSIONS

Treatment planning involves making choices about the treatment that is to be carried out. Knowledge of the options available, their uses, advantages and disadvantages, allows operator and patient to make informed choices about care. Having made the choice, the delivery of the chosen treatment can then be planned.

7 Organising care

How to deliver the agreed plan

Treatment priorities

Planning treatment
- Stabilisation phase
- Reassessment
- Restorative phase
- Continual maintenance, patient motivation and reassessment

Troubleshooting
- Loss of a temporary restoration
- Dental pain
- Tooth fracture
- Perforations
- Crown fracture
- Failure
- Denture problems
- Hypersensitivity

Perfect planning prevents pathetic performance!

HOW TO DELIVER THE AGREED TREATMENT PLAN

Having come to a diagnosis and made decisions and choices about treatment, it is now time to deliver the agreed treatment plan. You want the patient to understand what is being offered and this may be achieved in a number of ways. A verbal discussion may be adequate for a short, simple course of treatment, however it is a sensible precaution to provide a written plan in addition to the spoken word. It is well known that patients do not take in all the information we give them at appointments; so written advice is always a good approach. Some patients may find visual images easier to understand and a book of photographs of various treatment options can be a useful tool. More advanced forms of this approach include the use of diagnostic wax-ups, images from intra-oral, digital or Polaroid cameras and digitally enhanced images showing the before and after of proposed treatment.

A written treatment plan is important especially where treatment is complex, costly or when a patient needs more time to think about their care. In complex cases, a written treatment plan should not only be a list of treatment items, but also a timetable for the sequence in which treatment is to be delivered and the time intervals between items of care. This prepares the patient for what is involved in terms of time (and financial) commitments and allows them to plan their time for having dental care. It is always better to make appointments based on the longest possible times needed to allow for completion of the whole plan, as this can prevent the treatment plan getting out of control.

Not all treatment plans are straightforward or decided at the very outset of treatment. It may be that a staged approach will be required so that once teeth are investigated and the outcome known, then a further stage of treatment may be planned. This should be made clear to the patient at the outset.

Motivation of patients in respect of oral hygiene, diet management and smoking cessation are essential components of treatment and should be started at the early stage of treatment. This is where the team approach is essential. Dental hygienists play a key role in this stage of treatment as they can manage these elements of care very effectively and can provide excellent feedback on your patient's progress with this initial stage of care. Items of acute dental care can be carried out while the hygiene phase is taking place.

TREATMENT PRIORITIES

The first phase of treatment is the stabilisation phase. Acute conditions such as dental trauma, acute oral infections and dental pain should be dealt with as expeditiously as possible. This will not only give your patient confidence in your abilities to manage their problems, but will also allow you to assess how your patient responds to dental treatment. After the acute problems have been dealt with, it is time to put in place appropriate preventive measures. The key to any successful treatment is prevention of future disease. This may involve diet analysis and advice, oral hygiene measures, smoking cessation advice or the provision of a mouthguard for sports players. Iatrogenic factors such as ledges on restorations should be removed now to give good opportunity for periodontal health. Any non-surgical periodontal treatment should be started at this stage in those patients requiring this type of care. Teeth that are of hopeless prognosis and cannot be restored should be extracted early in the treatment plan to allow the tissues to heal. If you are unsure about the prognosis of a tooth, it is important to investigate it now and find out whether the tooth is restorable or whether it requires root canal treatment. Root canal treatment should be commenced at this stage and any failed restorations should be replaced and carious teeth restored. Finally, provisional prostheses such as immediate dentures or interim dentures should be provided.

After this initial stage, it is important to assess your patient's response to dental care and to reassess his/her dental condition. Some patients may never proceed beyond this stage, as they may not wish or be motivated to have further care. This may not be expressed explicitly but can be assessed by response to preventive measures. Such patients will stay in maintenance unless and until there is a more positive response to care. If there is a positive response, then the restorative phase of care can be carried out.

This stage involves continuing the preventive measures that were put in place in the stabilisation phase and providing definitive restorations. Before such restorations are provided it is important to ensure that you have all the information you require, such as articulated study casts and appropriate radiographs. Definitive restorations may involve root canal treatment, surgical periodontal treatment, inlays or onlays, crown and bridgework, definitive removable prostheses or implant retained restorations.

Obviously, not every patient requires all these steps and sometimes the order of treatment provision is changed because of patient priorities or emergency needs. However it is important to keep the overall aim of treatment in mind and not to be overtaken by events. All patients will require a suitable maintenance regime, involving reassessment and motivation, as appropriate for their oral condition, management skills, wants and needs.

PLANNING TREATMENT

Stabilisation phase

Acute conditions – pain, trauma, infection

Preventive measures – oral hygiene, diet control, sports guard, bite guard etc

Extraction of hopeless teeth

Removal of iatrogenic factors

Non surgical periodontal treatment

Restoration of carious teeth/treatment of failed restorations

Preliminary endodontics

Provisional prostheses

Reassessment

Usually at least six months later

Return to stabilisation phase or progress to restorative phase

Restorative phase

Continue preventive measures

Mounted study casts

Definitive endodontics

Surgical periodontal treatment

Crown and bridge work

Definitive prostheses

Continual maintenance, patient motivation and reassessment

TROUBLESHOOTING

Very few treatment plans run smoothly; even simple plans can develop problems. These may be related to individual teeth, the mouth overall or the patient. The common reasons for difficulties with a treatment plan relate to problems with individual teeth or items of treatment and because of this, it is important to have an overall aim for the treatment, because only in this way can you be sure that the plan will not be derailed by acute episodes.

Common dental problems that can arise during treatment include the following:

Loss of a temporary restoration

Patients should be advised to contact the dental surgery if this occurs, as the loss of a temporary restoration can increase the likelihood of pulp death, and can of course result in pain, poor appearance, gingival overgrowth, tooth drifting and overeruption, and loss of confidence in your care. An assessment should be made of the reason for temporary restoration loss so that the same mistake is not repeated in subsequent restorations. Failure may be caused by incorrect selection of initial restorative or luting material, leaving the restoration high on the occlusion or relying on the temporary restoration for an inappropriate time period.

Dental pain

Ideally an accurate diagnosis for dental pain should be made as soon as possible so that treatment decisions can be made. If you cannot come to an exact diagnosis, a provisional or differential diagnosis should be made so that interim or diagnostic treatment can be carried out. The pain may relate to the loss of a temporary restoration and the resulting exposed dentine or it may be pulpal inflammation following dental treatment on the now painful tooth. This may be reversible but if root treatment is required then this should be carried out, assuming that it is possible to restore the tooth, otherwise the tooth will have to be extracted. Root treatment is more difficult to carry out through crowns and therefore any tooth of doubtful pulpal prognosis should be very carefully assessed before crown provision. The prognosis of crown and bridge work is affected by the cutting of access cavities through the crown or bridge retainer. Root canal treatment after crown cementation often leads to fracture or failure of retention.

Tooth fracture

This may be the simple loss of an unsupported cusp in a tooth with a large restoration or a more complex fracture involving the pulp space. The latter is more common in root-treated teeth that have not had a restoration with cuspal coverage placed. If there is a complex fracture involving the pulp, there is little option but to extract the tooth. The same option applies if a vertical fracture of the root has occurred. Unfortunately this is not uncommon following post placement. If this involves an anterior tooth then a temporary, immediate denture or bridge will normally be provided.

Perforations

Perforations can occur during root canal treatment, pin placement or post preparation. If possible these should be repaired before the hole is made larger or further infection occurs. First an assessment should be made as to whether it will be possible to restore the tooth: if this is attainable then the perforation should be repaired with either mineral trioxide aggregate (MTA) or resin modified glass ionomer, depending on the size and position of the perforation.

Crown fracture

Fracture of a laboratory fabricated crown and its retaining core at gingival level can be restored in a number of ways. The quickest option is to place and lute a direct post (metal or fibre) in the canal, assuming the tooth is already root-filled. The old core is removed from the crown which is then filled with a chemically-cured resin core and luted in place. If the tooth is not root-filled then this treatment will have to be commenced to allow the crown to be retained by a post.

Failure

Failure of a restoration that is immediately adjacent to a partial denture component such as a clasp or rest seat can be difficult to manage, especially if a large restoration such as a crown is required. This can be achieved by taking the impression with the denture in place and sending the denture, in the impression, to the laboratory. However if the patient is reluctant to part with their denture then this technique is not possible. The laboratory can either pour the denture component of the impression in acrylic, rather than hard stone, or can create an acrylic coping which can be subsequently modified intra-orally.

Denture problems

Patients should, of course, be advised that new dentures might cause problems such as discomfort and speech difficulties. Following the insertion and fit of dentures, patients should be given a further review appointment so that initial problems with the denture can be resolved. Areas of discomfort may be caused by problems of fit or articulation. Speech problems may be due to poor adaptation or to incorrect tooth placement.

Hypersensitivity

Following items of dental treatment, patients may express concerns about dentine hypersensitivity. A careful history should be taken to ascertain whether this is the correct diagnosis, however this is not an uncommon concern following initial periodontal therapy and patients should be reassured about the cause. Treatment directed at occluding the dentinal tubules should be initiated.

Other Problems

Acute dental episodes are not the only reasons for problems occurring during a course of treatment. Patients may decline further treatment following the failure of local analgesia, tachycardia following injection of local anaesthetic solution containing adrenaline into a vessel, or fainting during a dental extraction. These episodes may result in your patient deciding that the risks associated with treatment are too great for them to manage.

Your initial assessment of the patient and their oral condition may have been incorrect and you may find that you cannot achieve your goal in relation to the patient's oral health. This can sometimes result in problems between you and your patient. Patients may change their mind about treatment and decide that they no longer wish to make the time or financial commitment required. Finally, you may find that you are no longer sure about the treatment you are carrying out. If this is the case, then you should stop and make a reassessment of the patient, their oral condition and your initial diagnosis and treatment plan.

8 | Continuing care

Maintenance programmes
- What to look for at check-ups
- How often to take radiographs
- Periodontal maintenance
- Dentures
- Crown and bridgework
- Tooth wear

Repair techniques
- Plastic restorations
- Crown and bridgework
- Dentures

Conclusion

MAINTENANCE PROGRAMMES

Diagnosis and treatment planning may take hours and treatment provision many months, but the ultimate success of our efforts is when the results are measured in decades by our patients. Restorations and their supporting tissues need active servicing to maintain a healthy state. Good communication is essential if an effective recall procedure is to be put into place. When a good dentist/patient rapport is present, patients are more likely to comply with maintenance advice. They are also more likely to communicate effectively at recall visits if they are relaxed and interested in their dental care. Sufficient time must be set aside for the recall appointment.

How often should patients be recalled for check-ups? There is little evidence to support a specific time interval for recall visits. Ideally, you should carry out a risk assessment exercise for each patient. This should take account of oral disease levels, past disease experience, restorations present, current disease patterns, lifestyle factors and medical history. Clinical judgement and knowledge of your patient are as important at this stage as they were at the diagnosis and planning stages.

What to look for at check-ups

Common items that apply to all patients should be reviewed in a systematic fashion. In general, you are looking for changes since you last saw the patient. This may be a change in their social or medical history, in their oral disease levels or in the condition of the restorations. Your history taking should concentrate on differences since the last visit. Clinical examinations should be in the context of the last examination: refer back to previous chartings and indices, special tests and radiographs, and look for changes in the soft and hard tissues, periodontium, teeth and restorations.

How often to take radiographs

Dental caries

Diagnostic yield for dental caries increases when bitewing radiographs are used in conjunction with the clinical examination. Caries activity is dependent upon interactions between plaque, tooth and sugar over time. It should be remembered that even in patients who are at high risk of caries, lesions may take three to four years to penetrate the approximal enamel.

The caries risk status should be assessed for each patient. To do this, the various risk factors for dental caries should be taken into account, namely the available clinical evidence, social and medical history, dietary habits, use of fluoride, plaque control and salivary factors. Patients who are at high risk of developing carious lesions should have bitewing radiographs taken at six-month intervals until no new or active lesions are apparent and the patient is no longer in a high risk category. Caries risk must be reassessed each time your patient is recalled. Low caries risk patients should have bitewings taken at two year intervals, or at even greater time intervals if there is evidence of continuing low caries risk. Again, this should be carefully assessed. Patients of medium risk should have annual bitewings, unless risk status alters. There are many ways that caries risk can change, for example it may be the result of diet changes following a change in social circumstances, or a reduction in salivary flow on prescription of certain drugs, or a patient becoming less dextrous at plaque removal.

Root-treated teeth

Radiographs are taken after root canal treatment in order to check for healing and to assess whether infection is present. Both the peak incidence of healing and the peak incidence of emerging chronic apical periodontitis are seen at one year. Almost 90 per cent of root-treated teeth that heal eventually demonstrate signs of healing at one year, and reversal of healing is rare. Radiographic follow-up at one year after completion of root canal treatment should be carried out. Teeth that have symptoms may require further follow-up. Cross-sectional studies have shown teeth that have been root-filled and subsequently restored with posts to have a higher failure rate than similar teeth without posts and therefore such teeth may also require additional radiographic follow-up.

Heavily restored teeth

With restorations come the risks of dental caries, periodontal, pulpal and periapical diseases. Many of these can be detected clinically, but radiographs can be an adjunct to this process. Higher diagnostic yields will be obtained if radiographic prescription is linked to symptoms and signs and to the type and size of restoration present. Radiographs of symptomless, vital teeth that have been crowned are more likely to reveal positive apical findings if taken in the two to ten years following cementation of the restoration.

Periodontal disease

Radiographs are secondary to clinical examination, even for the diagnosis of periodontal disease, and should only be taken after a thorough clinical examination has indicated their use as an adjunct. Bitewings offer the best detail and imaging geometry and as they are already indicated for caries assessment, they provide information about alveolar bone levels around teeth, without additional radiation dose. In cases where pocket measurements are greater than 6 mm, vertical bitewings should be prescribed. Radiographs are not used to monitor periodontal disease.

Periodontal maintenance

Maintaining periodontal health often requires considerable effort by the patient and the dental team. The aims of periodontal maintenance are to control dental plaque and prevent further loss of periodontal support. A practical routine for periodontal maintenance should include:

- Examination and evaluation of the periodontal conditions by measurement of clinical attachment levels, assessment of bleeding and gingival inflammation and possibly radiographic examination of any teeth with signs or symptoms.
- Evaluation of the patient's level of plaque control.
- Renewed motivation, oral hygiene instruction, elimination of calculus and other plaque traps and professional cleaning of the teeth.
- Treatment of any recurrence of the periodontal disease.

The frequency of maintenance visits will depend on the patient's level of plaque control, the number of plaque retentive features and the patient's disease susceptibility. Recall periods will normally be between three months and one year.

Dentures

The aim in denture maintenance is to ensure that oral health, comfort, function and appearance are preserved despite changes in the supporting tissues and in the dentures. Partial denture wearers have more plaque, root surface caries and cervical restorations than patents without partial dentures. Residual ridges may also change shape. This may be rapid in the first year of denture wearing and can continue at an average of 1mm per annum over the next few years, particularly in those patients whose dentures are mainly mucosal borne. The position of the denture on the tissues is modified by this change in ridge shape and the resultant loss of fit and the change in the occlusal balance can result in soft tissue trauma and inflammation. Wear of the acrylic teeth can also alter the occlusal balance and this may encourage further alveolar bone resorption. Denture trauma can contribute to chronic atrophic candidiasis (denture stomatitis) and denture hyperplasia.

Regular maintenance for denture-wearing patients is obviously very important. A practical routine for denture maintenance should include:
- Examination and evaluation of the edentulous areas and of the dentures by assessment of their stability and retention, peripheral extensions, occlusion and smooth surfaces;
- Evaluation of the patient's level of denture hygiene measures and plaque control;
- Assessment of caries levels, especially at cervical margins and on any root abutments for overdentures;
- Renewed motivation and oral and denture hygiene instruction, including fluoride application to overdenture abutments;
- Treatment of any denture problems by peripheral or occlusal adjustment, relining, copying or replacing.

Crown and bridgework

Maintaining crown and bridgework requires manual dexterity by the patient and careful, regular examination by the dental team. The aims of crown and bridge maintenance are to control biological factors such as dental caries and prevent mechanical failures such as cementation failure. The latter is most likely to occur in the first twelve months following cementation.

A practical routine for crown and bridge maintenance should include:
- Examination and evaluation of the periodontal conditions and the patient's level of plaque and dietary control (as above);
- Renewed motivation, oral hygiene instruction especially interproximally and under pontics, elimination of calculus and other plaque traps and professional cleaning of the teeth;
- Examination for cementation failure of bridgework by looking for fluid movement/bubbles at the cervical margins;

- Porcelain fracture or wear should be assessed and then polished or repaired with resin composite directly or with an indirect porcelain veneer. Alternatively, the restoration may need to be replaced to satisfy aesthetic requirements;
- Radiographs should be taken using the suggested selection criteria (see fig. 2.7).

On completion of extensive anterior crown and bridgework it may be prudent to supply the patient with a mouthguard to protect the restorations, especially if the patient plays contact sports.

Tooth wear

The aetiology of the tooth wear, if identified, and the subsequent management of the wear will define the maintenance programme. Patients with tooth wear may be concerned about appearance, sensitivity or they may wish information about the long term prognosis for their teeth.

A practical routine for maintenance of tooth wear patients should include:

- Examination and evaluation of the tooth wear by assessing symptoms such as sensitivity and signs such as stain collection or whether restorations are proud of the remaining tooth or are worn. Comparison with previous stone models, photographs, or impression material indices may also be used.
- Renewed motivation, and assessment of the patient's grinding or brushing habits and dietary control.
- Careful checking of the medical and social history.
- Radiographs should be taken using the suggested selection criteria (see above).
- Use of sensitive formula toothpaste, fluoride or occluding agents to manage any sensitivity problems.

REPAIR TECHNIQUES

Failure can be difficult to define. What one dentist or an individual patient considers to be less than ideal may be different from another dentist or patient. This is not necessarily wrong, but is a variation in judgement. In general dental practice, more than half of the dentists' time is spent in replacing restorations that have been assessed to have failed. Failure may be mechanical, in that the restorative material has failed, biological as the result of further disease or a combination of both mechanical and biological failure. The reasons for failure of any restoration should be carefully assessed to avoid repetition of the same error, if possible.

Plastic restorations

When restorations are replaced the cavity will increase in size, however carefully the previous material is removed. The longevity for amalgam and composite restorations decreases as the size of the cavity increases. The pulp will also become 'stressed' by the assaults of dental disease and restoration placement. It is important to make an accurate diagnosis of the reason for restoration failure and consider methods of repair – rather than replace complete restorations, a more preservative approach is to repair the deficiency or refurbish the restoration. Repair may be with a different material, such as a fissure sealant resin or a flowable resin composite. Ultra small burs or air abrasion can be used to remove the areas of stain or caries before the material is applied. A worn or fractured surface may also be repaired if the area is freshened with a bur or air abrasion before the resin composite is applied.

Crowns and bridges

Small marginal gaps or early carious lesions at the margins may be repaired in a similar manner to repairing plastic restorations, namely careful and minimal removal of any diseased tissues and replacement with flowable resin composite or glass ionomer type materials. Fractured porcelain may be repaired with direct resin composite and bonding systems that include coupling agents to achieve a bond to the ceramic and/or metal. Larger fractures may be repaired by luting a porcelain veneer to the prepared fracture area.

Dentures

Dentures with fractured components may be repaired or modified, usually in the laboratory. Dentures that no longer fit may be refurbished by relining or rebasing at the chairside or in the laboratory. Worn occlusal surfaces can be built up with cold cure acrylic to assess patient tolerance of the changed occlusal vertical dimension before replacement dentures are provided.

CONCLUSION

Effective recall and maintenance protocols and the ability to repair restorations to increase their acceptable clinical longevity are essential aspects of successful dental practice. If appropriate diagnostic, management and treatment decisions were made at the start of care then maintenance should, in general, be a predictable procedure.

9 Treatment planning examples

CASE 1 – STEPHEN

Introduction

This patient is a 31-year-old male who works as a manual labourer. He wants to face up to the dentist after a previous bad experience – his fear of dental treatment is so great that he has extracted two of his teeth with pliers. He used to smoke 20 cigarettes a day for 15 years but gave up eight months ago. He has not drunk alcohol for two years. He is separated and has a young son.

Presenting complaint

Stephen was hit in the face approximately 18 months ago and following that noticed that his anterior teeth were mobile. He came to the dentist with generalised low grade pain from all areas of his mouth.

Medical history

The patient is fit and well. He has no allergies and is not taking any medication from his doctor.

Extra-oral examination

No abnormalities found.

Intra-oral examination

Angles class III incisor relationship
Generalised plaque and calculus
Gingival tissues red and inflamed
Mobility of the upper anterior teeth at the Grade I–II level
Caries present
  UR6 mesial
  UL6 occlusal
  UL7 occlusal
  LL6 distal

Charting (fig. 9.1)

Basic periodontal examination

2	3	3
2	3	2

Radiographs

A Dental Panoramic Tomogram (DPT) (fig. 9.2) was taken when the patient first attended. This showed a horizontal pattern of periodontal bone loss. There were retained roots in the UR8 and UL5 regions. The small retained root fragments at LR8 and LL7 had exfoliated spontaneously between the patient's first and second attendances.

Diet record

A three day diet record was completed by the patient (fig. 9.3). The patient was not deemed to be a high caries risk and the few sugar intakes that he has seemed to be restricted to meal times. He does not take sugar in his tea.

Gingival bleeding scores

Baseline score 72%
After three months 51%

Plaque scores

Baseline score 78%
After three months 53%

Diagnosis

- Chronic periodontitis
- Retained roots UR8, UL5
- Caries UR6, UL6, UL7, LL6
- Dental anxiety

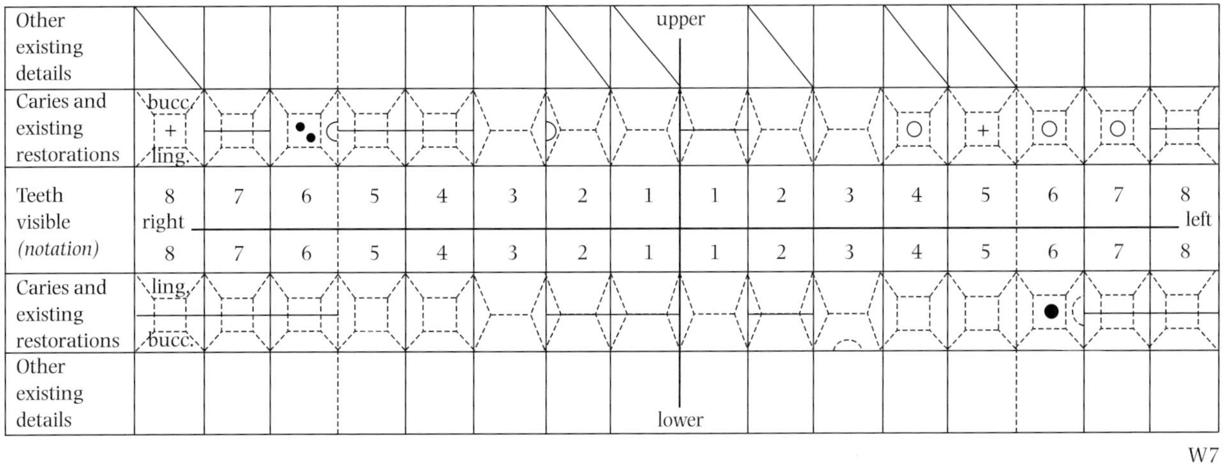

Teeth charting (upper)

	Right															Left
Other existing details																
Caries and existing restorations	bucc/ +/ling															
Teeth visible (notation)	8	7	6	5	4	3	2	1	1	2	3	4	5	6	7	8
	8	7	6	5	4	3	2	1	1	2	3	4	5	6	7	8
Caries and existing restorations	ling/ /bucc															
Other existing details																

upper / lower

W7

Figure 9.1. Case 1 charting.

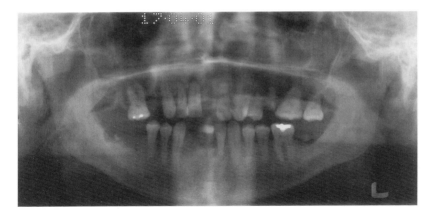

Figure 9.2. Case 1 DPT radiograph.

Day 1	0630 Bowl of cereal, three slices of toast, one cup of tea
	1000 One ham sandwich, one mug of tea
	1300 Curry, chips and rice, one can of Coke
	1800 Roast chicken, potatoes, carrots, cabbage, gravy
	2200 Cheese on toast, one mug of tea
Day 2	0630 Bowl of cereal, three slices of toast, one cup of tea
	1000 One egg and two slices of bacon on toast, two mugs of tea
	1300 Beef salad sandwich, two doughnuts, one mug of tea
	1730 Pizza and chips
	2200 Tea and toast
Day 3	1100 Bacon, Sausage, egg, mushroom, fried bread, toast, tea
	1500 Roast lamb, potatoes, carrots, cabbage, gravy, apple pie
	1900 Kentucky Fried Chicken, two cans of Coke
	2230 Tea and toast

Figure 9.3. Stephen's diet diary.

Treatment plan

Stabilisation

- Supra- and subgingival scaling
- Oral hygiene instruction
- Diet advice
- Desensitisation to treatment – the patient had had a traumatic experience having a general anaesthetic for dental extractions as a child. Before having any further extractions, he asked to be taken to where he had had a general anaesthetic previously. He felt that seeing the area would help him to come to terms with his anxiety.

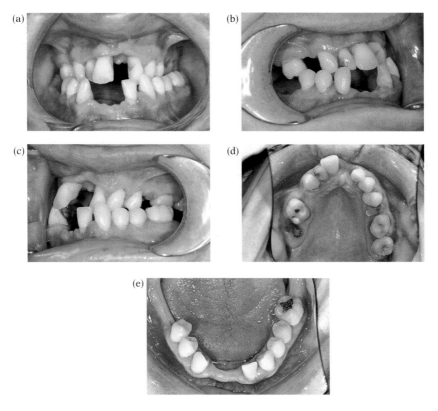

Figure 9.4. (a) Pre-treatment anterior view. (b) Pre-treatment right lateral view. (c) Pre-treatment left lateral view. (d) Pre-treatment upper occlusal view. (e) Pre-treatment lower occlusal view.

Definitive treatment
- Restore UR6 with composite resin
- Restore UL6 and UL7 with amalgam
- Extract retained roots at UR8 and UL5
- Construct upper and lower partial immediate dentures
- Extract UR2, UR1, UL2, UL4 and LL2 and fit immediate dentures

Maintenance
- Watch early carious lesion at LL6
- Reinforce oral hygiene instruction and diet advice
- Review extraction sites for resorption and check the fit of the immediate dentures. Consider replacement dentures if necessary.

COMMENTARY

This is a simple case in terms of the treatment provided but it involved a considerable amount of time and care. A gentle patient-centred approach

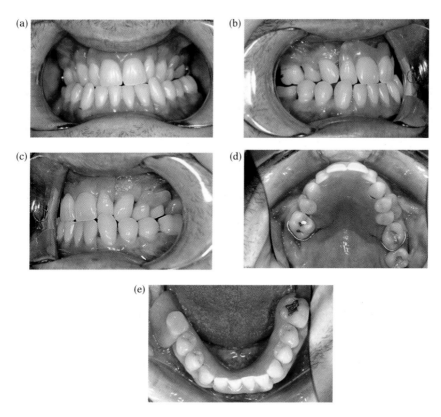

Figure 9.5. (a) Post-treatment anterior view with dentures. (b) Post-treatment right lateral view with dentures. (c) Post-treatment left lateral view with dentures. (d) Post-treatment upper occlusal view with dentures. (e) Post-treatment lower occlusal view with dentures.

was used, with treatment proceeding at a pace determined by the patient. To overcome anxiety regarding local anaesthesia, topical anaesthetic cream was always used to make injections as painless as possible. An excellent aesthetic and functional result has been achieved and the patient has been successfully reintroduced to dental treatment. It is hoped that he will now attend a general dental practitioner on a regular basis.

CASE 2 – ROBIN

Introduction

This patient is a 30-year-old single male who works full time as an air steward. He smokes approximately 20 cigarettes per day and consumes an average amount of alcohol. He does not have his own dentist but has had complex treatment in the past. He brushes his teeth twice a day and uses floss. He presented because the metal ceramic crown on UR1 was fractured on the palatal surface.

Presenting complaint

He was unhappy with the appearance of his teeth. He had noticed the poor appearance of the crowns about one year ago when the crown margins became evident. The crowns were approximately 6–8 years old. He had no pain but some gingival recession and bleeding on brushing.

Medical history

The patient is fit and well. He has no allergies and is not taking any medication from his doctor.

Extra-oral examination

No abnormalities found.

Intra-oral examination

Angles class II Division I occlusion with lower incisor crowding
Generalised plaque and calculus
Staining of the teeth due to smoking
Gingival tissues in upper anterior region red and inflamed
Crown margins deficient on UR5, UR1, UL1, UL2 and LL5
Large amalgam restorations in the upper first premolars showing on buccal aspect
Recurrent caries in UR3 and LL8
Minimal enamel caries LL3
Stained margins of composite restorations on UR3 and UL3
Deficient lingual aspect of composite restoration LL3

Charting (fig. 9.6)

Basic periodontal examination

2	3	2
3	2	2

Radiographs (fig. 9.7)

Left and right bitewings
Periapical views of the upper and lower anterior teeth and UR5, UR4, LL4, LL5, LL8.
These showed that UR5 had an orthograde root filling present. There was slight widening of the apical periodontal ligament but it was not possible to determine whether this was a stable or deteriorating situation.

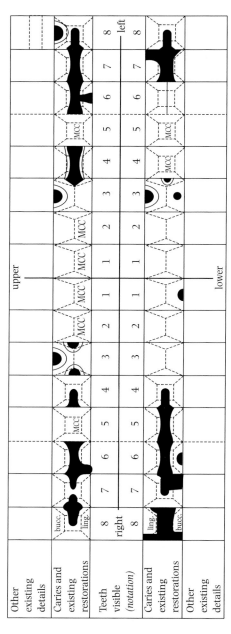

Figure 9.6. Case 2 charting.

W7

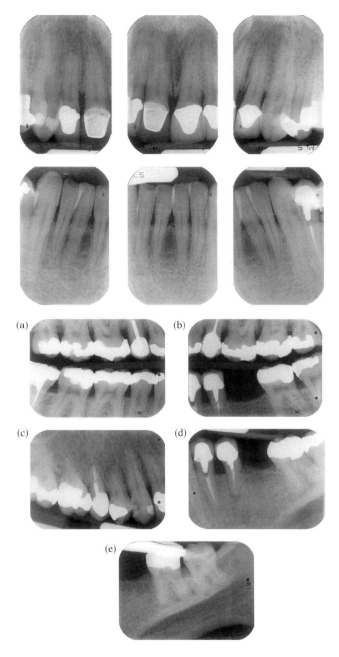

(a) (b)

(c) (d)

(e)

Figure 9.7. Case 2 radiographs (radiograph (e) was taken in mid-treatment when LL8 had a temporary restoration in place of the previous MO amalgam restoration).

The LL5 had an orthograde root filling present. There was slight widening of the periodontal ligament space.

The LL8 had recurrent caries but no apical pathology was present.

Vitality testing

UR4 – no response

LL8 – positive response

Gingival bleeding scores

Baseline score 41%

After one month 16%

After five months 11%

Plaque scores

Baseline score 33%

After one month 18%

After five months 12%

Diagnosis

- Chronic periodontitis
- Chronic apical periodontitis LL5
- Deficient crown margins UR5, UR1, UL1, UL2 and LL5
- Poor aesthetic appearance UR4, UR3, UR2, UL3 and UL4
- Deficient restoration LL3
- Recurrent caries LL8 and UR3
- Enamel caries LR3
- Plaque retention factors (overhanging margins) UR6 and UL7

Treatment plan

Stabilisation

- Supra- and subgingival scaling
- Oral hygiene instruction
- Diet advice and smoking cessation advice
- Removal of plaque retention factors UR6 and UL7
- Monitor buccal cervical lesion LR3

Definitive treatment

- Redo endodontic treatment on LL5
- Restore UR3, UL3, UL4 and LL3 with composite resin
- Full gold crown LL8
- Post-retained metal-ceramic crowns UR5 and LL5

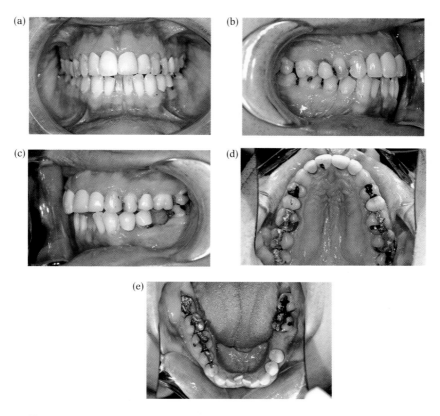

Figure 9.8. (a) Pre-treatment anterior view. (b) Pre-treatment right lateral view. (c) Pre-treatment left lateral view. (d) Pre-treatment upper occlusal view. (e) Pre-treatment lower occlusal view.

- Metal-ceramic crowns UR2, UR1, UL1 and UL2
- Alteration to the treatment plan:
- A fracture was found in the UR4 from the mesial to the distal surfaces. The pulp was necrotic. Root canal treatment was carried out on UR4 followed by a metal-ceramic crown.

Maintenance

Review oral hygiene and reiterate diet and smoking cessation advice

COMMENTARY

This patient had a heavily restored mouth for someone of his age. His main concern was aesthetics as his job as an airline steward brings him into close proximity to the general public. The amalgam restorations in the upper first

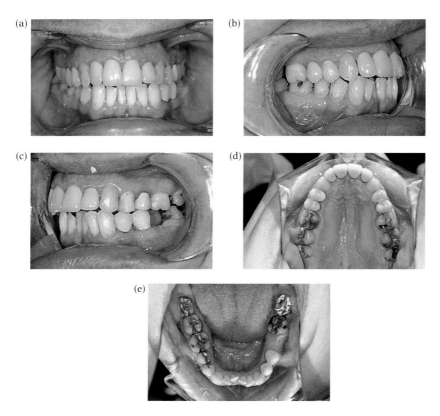

Figure 9.9. (a) Post-treatment anterior view. (b) Post-treatment right lateral view. (c) Post-treatment left lateral view. (d) Post-treatment upper occlusal view. (e) Post-treatment lower occlusal view.

premolars were particularly noticeable. By replacing some of his amalgam restorations with composite and replacing the upper metal-ceramic crowns with a shade and contour more in keeping with the remaining teeth, a good aesthetic improvement has been achieved.

Direct composite has been used in the upper canines. One must always remember that any restoration has a definite lifespan, whether it be a direct or indirect restoration, and in a patient of this age one must plan for the long-term regarding replacement restorations. Crowns are always an option for the canines in the future if necessary.

CASE 3 – PATRICIA

Introduction

This patient is a 55-year-old married female who works part-time as a bank clerk. She attends regularly for treatment and is well motivated.

She gave up smoking 20 years ago and drinks approximately 10 units of alcohol per week.

Presenting complaint

She had lost a crown in the lower left quadrant and complained that her upper and lower partial dentures were loose. The present dentures were approximately 10 years old. They are unretentive and unstable. Last year the patient had new dentures constructed but has been unable to wear them and they were very uncomfortable. The crown was lost approximately one year ago.

Medical history

The patient has osteoarthritis in her hips. She is allergic to Penicillin.

Extra-oral examination

No abnormalities found

Intra-oral examination

Upper partial denture unstable, rocking laterally
Lower partial denture very unretentive

Charting (fig. 9.10)
Basic periodontal examination

–	2	–
–	2	2

Radiographs (fig. 9.11)

Periapical radiographs were taken of UL3, UL5, LL4 and LL5

Gingival bleeding scores

Baseline score 6%
After two months 12%
After three months 6%

Plaque scores

Baseline score 42%
After two months 29%
After three months 31%

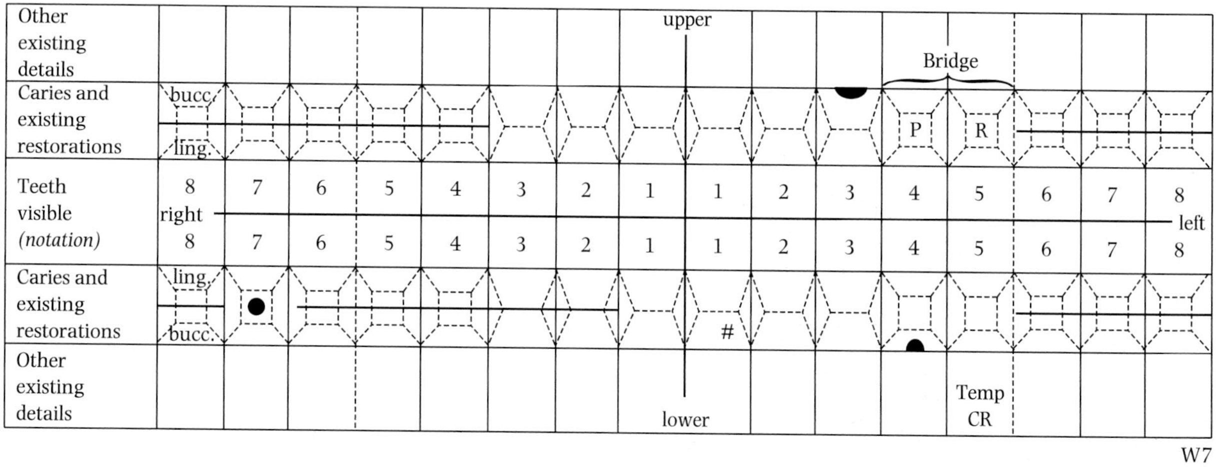

Figure 9.10. Case 3 charting.

Other existing details																
Caries and existing restorations	bucc. / ling.															
Teeth visible (*notation*)	8	7	6	5	4	3	2	1	1	2	3	4	5	6	7	8
	8	7	6	5	4	3	2	1	1	2	3	4	5	6	7	8
Caries and existing restorations	ling. / bucc.															
Other existing details																

right — upper — left

lower

Bridge P R

Temp CR

#

W7

(a)

(b) (c)

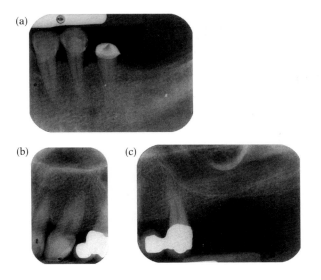

Figure 9.11. Case 3 radiographs.

Diagnosis

- Plaque-induced gingivitis
- Unretentive crown LL5 with insufficient crown height remaining
- Unretentive and unstable upper and lower partial dentures

Treatment plan

Stabilisation

- Supra- and subgingival scaling
- Oral hygiene instruction with brush and floss

Definitive treatment

- Elective endodontic treatment LL5
- Rhine precision attachment LL5
- New upper and lower partial cobalt chrome dentures

Maintenance

Review oral hygiene including denture hygiene

Denture design

Upper denture

Rest seats   UR3 and UL3 cingulum rests (cast cobalt chrome)
              UL5 distal occlusal rest (cast cobalt chrome)

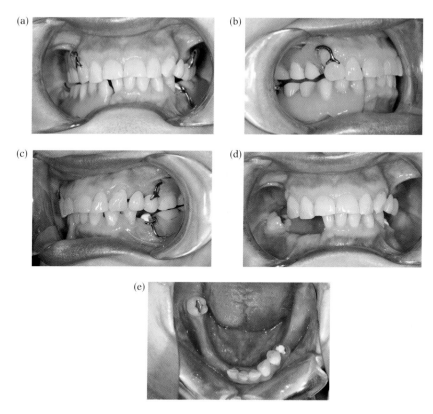

Figure 9.12. (a) Pre-treatment anterior view with dentures. (b) Pre-treatment right lateral view with dentures. (c) Pre-treatment left lateral view with dentures. (d) Pre-treatment anterior view without dentures. (e) Pre-treatment lower occlusal view without denture.

Clasps	UR3 gingivally approaching 'I' bar (cast cobalt chrome)
	UL5 gingivally approaching 'I' bar (cast cobalt chrome)
Connector	Cobalt chrome anterior and posterior palatal bars

Lower denture

Rest seats	LL4 distal occlusal rest (cast cobalt chrome)
Clasps	LR7 circumferential clasp (cast cobalt chrome)
	LL4 gingivally approaching 'I' bar (cast cobalt chrome)
Attachment	Rhine precision attachment LL5
Connector	Cobalt chrome lingual plate

COMMENTARY

This patient had dentures, which had been constructed only one year previously, but she was unable to wear them. In addition, the crown on the LL5

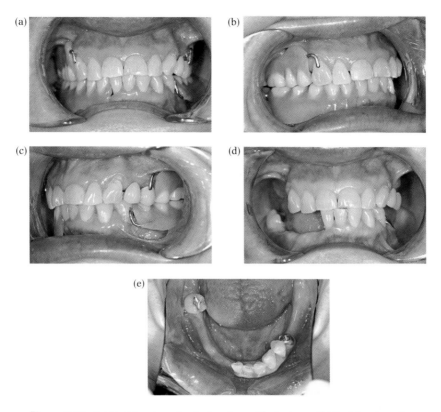

Figure 9.13. (a) Post-treatment anterior view with dentures. (b) Post-treatment right lateral view with dentures. (c) Post-treatment left lateral view with dentures. (d) Post-treatment anterior view without dentures. (e) Post-treatment lower occlusal view without denture.

had come off. From a clinical and radiographic examination, it was clear that the LL5 had insufficient coronal tooth tissue to support a crown but in addition, this crown was being used as a retentive abutment for a lower partial denture. This combination of factors lead to the failure of the crown at LL5. Rather than repeating the same mistake, an alternative approach has been taken. Elective endodontic treatment is an option where there is insufficient coronal tooth tissue to support a crown. If the root is of adequate size, it may be possible to construct a post-retained crown once the endodontic treatment has been successfully completed. In this case the root was short and a post-retained crown was not an option. However, the root has been successfully used to retain a precision attachment which increases the retention of the lower partial denture without overloading the abutment. A retention clasp is also present on LL4 which means that the precision attachment is not the only retentive element in that quadrant.

CASE 4 – IRENE

Introduction

Irene is 38 years old, married and works shifts as an emergency room assistant in a local teaching hospital. She is an irregular attender to the dental surgery, although she has had dental treatment including crowns in the past. Her social history revealed that she smokes 20 cigarettes aday.

Presenting complaint

She presented with a fractured tooth in the upper left quadrant which is not causing her any pain. She also reported that her gums bleed.

Medical history

Prozac
Hormone replacement therapy (HRT)

Extra-oral examination

Nothing abnormal detected

Intra-oral examination

Discoloured and carious UL3
Acrylic, mucosal borne partial upper denture – 20 years old and replacing
   UR6 UR5 UL2 UL5 UL6
Soft tissues under partial denture are inflamed
Generalised plaque and subgingival calculus deposits
Minimal pocketing, bleeding on probing
Multiple carious lesions

Charting (fig. 9.14)
Basic periodontal examination

–	2	3
2	2	2

Special investigations

Periapicals of the crowned teeth and teeth with large carious lesions i.e. UR2
   UL1 UL3 LR4 LL5
Diet sheet
Vitality tests of the discoloured UL3 and the carious LR4 and LL5

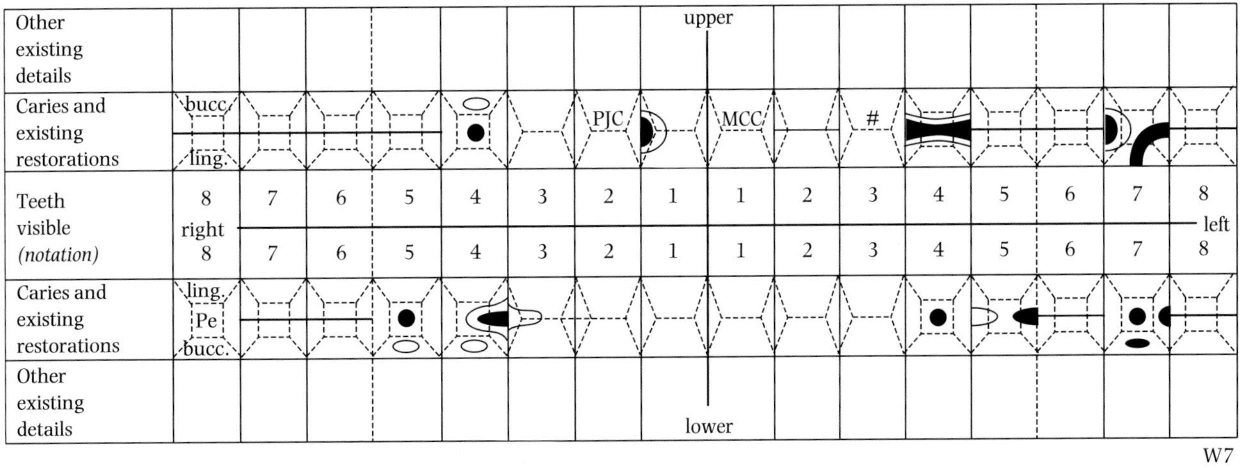

Dental charting grid (rotated in original):

Other existing details																
Caries and existing restorations (bucc. / ling.)																
Teeth visible (notation)	8	7	6	5	4	3	2	1	1	2	3	4	5	6	7	8
	8	7	6	5	4	3	2	1	1	2	3	4	5	6	7	8
Caries and existing restorations (ling. / Pe / bucc.)																
Other existing details																

right — upper — left
lower

PJC   MCC   #

W7

Figure 9.14. Case 4 charting.

DAY Friday | DAY Saturday

TIME	FOOD	QUANTITY	TIME	FOOD	QUANTITY
10.30 am	Toast—flora margarine Tea—2 tspn sugar	1 slice 1 beaker	6.30 am	Toast—Flora margarine Tea—2 tspn sugar	1 slice 1 beaker
11.30 am	Tea—2 tspn sugar Digestive biscuit	1 beaker 1 biscuit (low fat)	8.30 am	Toast—strawberry jam Tea—2 tspn sugar	1 slice 1 beaker
3.30 pm	Yoghurt—low fat with fruit		3.15 pm	Cheese muffin Tea—2 tspn sugar	$\frac{1}{2}$ muffin thin slice cheese 1 beaker
between 2.45–9.15 pm	Tic Tac mints	$\frac{1}{2}$ packet approx 20 mints	5 pm	Tea 2 tspn sugar Digestive biscuit	1 beaker 1 biscuit (low fat)
10 pm	Tea—2 tspn sugar	1 beaker	7 pm	Tea—2 tspn sugar Digestive biscuit	1 beaker 1 biscuit (low fat)
11 pm	Toast—flora margarine Tea—2 tspn sugar	2 slices 1 beaker	9 pm	Pizza—chicken 1 Sweetcorn topping coleslaw	$\frac{1}{2}$ 9-inch pizza
11.45 pm	Tea-2 tspn sugar Digestive biscuit	1 beaker 1 biscuit (low fat)		Tea—2 tspn sugar	1 beaker
			11 pm	Tea—2 tspn sugar Digestive biscuit	1 beaker 1 biscuit (low fat)

Figure 9.15. Irene's diet diary.

Diagnosis

- Chronic atrophic candidiasis (denture stomatitis)
- Plaque induced gingivitis
- Edentulous saddles
- Non-vital UL3, LL5
- Caries in UR4 UL3 UL4 UL7 LL5 LR3 LR4 LR5 related to frequent sugar intakes
- Poorly contoured restorations UR2 UR1 UL1
- Ill-fitting, worn partial upper denture
- Partially erupted LR8

Treatment plan

Stabilisation phase

- Diet analysis and advice
- Denture hygiene advice and topical antifungal agents
- Tooth brushing instruction and scaling and polishing
- Root canal treatment of UL3 and LL5
- Amalgams UL6 LL5 LR4
- Composites LR3 LR 4 LR5 UR1 UR4

Restorative phase

- Replacement metal ceramic crowns UR2 and UL1
- Conventional cantilever bridge UL2 (pontic) UL3 (retainer)
- Flossing and interdental brush use, especially around crowns and bridge

Maintenance phase

- Reinforcement of dietary advice and oral hygiene measures
- Caries assessment
- Monitor partially erupted LR8

COMMENTARY

Irene's diet diary revealed a very frequent sugar intake, mainly in tea and in the form of mint sweets, consumed between meals. Dietary advice centred on the use of sugar substitutes in tea and sugar-free mints rather than conventional mints.

Denture hygiene advice and various topical antifungal agents were unsuccessful in resolving the chronic atrophic candidiasis (denture stomatitis) because Irene eventually confessed that she never took her denture out and that her husband was unaware that she wore a denture. Her reason for wearing the denture was because it replaced the missing UL2. In order to get the inflammation to resolve, an interim bridge was made to replace the UL2

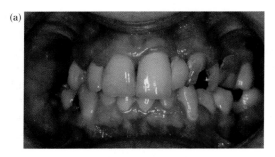

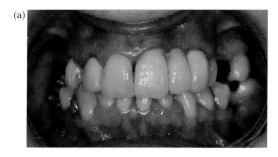

Figure 9.16. Before.

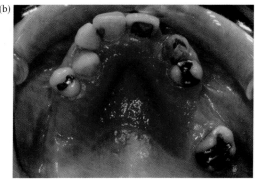

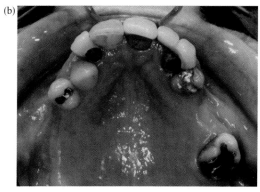

Figure 9.17. After.

during the stabilisation phase of the treatment plan. The temporary bridge was of conventional type cantilevered from UL1 (already crowned and due for replacement of the crown owing to recurrent caries). The permanent bridge was cantilevered from the UL3 as the UL1 was restored with a post-retained crown and it was decided that the prognosis for the bridge was better if the UL3 were used as the abutment tooth, as this tooth was not restored with a post.

The restorative phase of treatment was only carried out many months after completion of the stabilisation phase, as it would have been inappropriate to provide complex restorative care for a patient with an unstable oral condition (figs 9.16 and 9.17).

References and further reading

GATHERING INFORMATION

Corah NL, Gale EH, Illig S. Assessment of a dental anxiety scale. *J Am Dent Assoc* 1978; 97: 816–819.

Humphris GM, Morrison T, Lindsay SJE. The Modified Dental Anxiety Scale: validation and United Kingdom norms. *Community Dental Health* 1995; 12: 143–150.

Smith BGN, Knight JK. An index for measuring the wear of teeth. *Br Dent J* 1984; 156: 435–438.

Speilberger CD, Gorsuch RL, Lushene RE. *STAI Manual for the State-Trait Inventory*. Palo Alto, California: Consulting Psychologists Press, 1970.

Vrana S, McNeil D, McGlynn DA. A structured interview for assessing dental fear. *J Behav Ther Exp Psychiatry* 1986; 17: 175–178.

PATIENT MANAGEMENT

Kent G. Memory of dental pain. *Pain* 1985; 21(2): 187–194.

North West Medicines Information Centre. *Surgical Management of the Primary Care Dental Patient on Warfarin*. July 2001. Available from North West Medicines Information Centre, Pharmacy Practice Unit, 70 Pembroke Place, Liverpool L69 3GF.

Albandar JM, Streckfus CF, Adesanya MR, Winn DM. Cigar, pipe and cigarette smoking as risk factors for periodontal disease and tooth loss. *J Perio* 2000; 71(12): 1874–1881.

Jansson L, Lavstedt S, Frithiof L, Theobald H. Relationship between oral health and mortality in cardiovascular diseases. *J Clin Perio* 2001; 28(8): 762–768.

Kinane DF. Causation and pathogenesis of periodontal disease. *Periodontology* 2000; 25: 8–20.

Kleinknecht RA, Bernstein DA. The assessment of dental fear. *Behav Ther* 1978; 9: 626–634.

Locker D. *An Introduction to Behavioural Science and Dentistry*. 1989; London: Routledge.

Mellor AC. Dental anxiety and attendance in the North-West of England. *J Dent* 1992; 20: 207–210.

REACHING A DIAGNOSIS

Ekstrand KR, Ricketts DNJ, Kidd EAM. Occlusal caries: pathology, diagnosis and logical management. *Dent Update* 2001; 28: 380–387.

DECISION-MAKING

Downie RS, Macnaughton J. *Clinical Judgement: Evidence In Practice*. 2000; Oxford: Oxford University Press.

Kay EJ, Blinkhorn AS. Some factors related to dentists' decisions to extract teeth. *Community Dental Health* 1987; 4: 3–8.

Kay EJ, Nuttall NM. *Clinical Decision Making: An Art Or A Science?* 1997; London: BDJ Books.

Lambden P (ed.). *Dental Law And Ethics.* 2002; Oxford: Radcliffe Medical Press.

CLINICAL CHOICES

Kidd EAM, Joyston-Bechal S. *Essentials Of Dental Caries.* 1997; Oxford: Oxford University Press.

Wassell RW, Steele JG, Walls AWG. *A Clinical Guide To Crowns And Other Extra-Coronal Restorations.* 2002; London: BDJ Books.

CONTINUING CARE

Nuttall N, Steele JG, Nunn J *et al. A Guide To The UK Adult Dental Health Survey 1998.* 2001; London: BDJ Books.

Index